Health through inner body cleansing

Health through inner body cleansing

The famous MAYR intestinal therapy from Europe

Erich Rauch, M. D.

With 15 illustrations and 2 tables

Translated by Mollie Comerford Peters

4th English Edition

HAUG

Editions HAUG INTERNATIONAL · Brussels

Rauch, Erich:
Health through inner body cleansing : the famous Mayr intestinal therapy from Europe / Erich Rauch. Transl. by Mollie Commerford Peters. – 4th Engl. ed. – Brussels, Belgium : Editions HAUG INTERNATIONAL, 1993.
ISBN 2-8043-4009-0

Printing history: 1st–39th German edition 1957–1992

Editions HAUG INTERNATIONAL
Chaussée de Ninove 1072
B-1080 Bruxelles/Brussels

2nd edition 1988
3rd edition 1990
4th edition 1993

Titel-No. 4009 · ISBN 2-8043-4009-0

Dépôt légal: Bibliothèque Royale de Belgique
n° D/1993/6159/05

Imprimé: Progressdruck GmbH, 6720 Speyer
Federal Republic of Germany

Contents

Part I
Illness and Health — a New View

Part II
Recovery by the Mayr Plan

Part III
Better nutrition and a healthier way of life

Many physicians in Austria, Germany, Holland and Belgium are currently using the Mayr method in their practice. Extremely serious illnesses, such malignancies and infectious diseases like TB and AIDS, are **not** treated with this therapy. Persons who are chronically underweight, those suffering from hyperthyroidism or persons with serious mental illness cannot be treated by this therapy either. On the other hand, the following indications have been successfully treated:

Digestive disturbances such as constipation, dyspepsia (indigestion), stomach, liver, gallbladder and intestinal complaints; poor blood profiles (lipids, high cholesteral, uric acid, etc.); **obesity** and all its **attendant risks**, heart problems, Type II diabetes, and back problems; rheumatism and gout. The close link between **attractiveness and good digestion** means that Mayr treatment can also be considered an "inner beauty treatment" or "natural cosmetic aid" and diet plan. People who are obese usually lose a significant amount of weight and end up with a good ratio of body fat to muscle. But above all, Mayr therapy offers the modern citizen a **natural preventive and regenerative treatment** for body and soul.

The cartoonist who drew the following pictures has somewhat humorously captured the experience of going through Mayr therapy at a health spa:

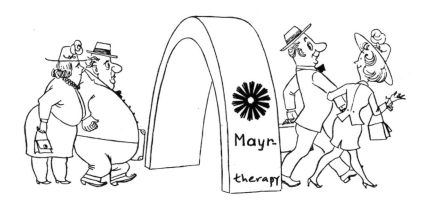

A physician schooled in the Mayr method and a positive attitude on the part of the patient are prerequisites to successful therapy. The supervising physician can make going through Mayr therapy much easier for most people and even make it an enjoyable experience. Psychological help is also available to people who lack the necessary will power. Our cartoonist has given us a somewhat exaggerated illustration of this point:

"You should know right from the start that this is the only exit from our health spa ..."

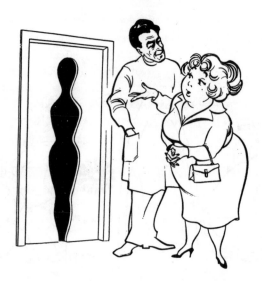

Foreword to the 30th edition*

The discoveries *F. X. Mayr* made are gradually becoming more accepted. Up until his death at the age of 90 (1965) he was unusually active and mentally alert, and personally showed his appreciation and approval of this work, both orally and in writing. How happy he would have been about the spread of his teachings, how they found expression in the growing number of translations of this book and the appearance of its 30th edition in German! Several hundred thousand readers, among them many physicians, have now studied its contents and in many cases adopted its precepts. Since this small book alone could not meet all the special needs of contemporary, affluent society, it was followed by other writings: "Cleansing the Blood and Other Bodily Fluids", which lays the foundation for natural medical treatment and introduces moderate elimination therapy, *F. X. Mayr's* mildest form of treatment; "Moderate Elimination Diet", which appeared still later includes recipes for easily digestible dishes and offers guidelines for better nutrition. Fulfilling a genuine need, "Curing Colds and Infections Naturally" was also published. It has long since proven its worth, as attested to by letters of success and gratitude from all over the world, especially from mothers with children prone to infections. Natural cures are more important today than ever because the basic health and powers of resistance of many children and adults have been significantly reduced due to the widespread use of high dosage drugs, especially for treating infections, and may even affect the success of *Mayr* therapies.

Training courses for physicians in Dr. *Mayr's* diagnostics and therapy have been very successful and have sparked increasing interest. The booklet "Diagnostics According to *F. X. Mayr*", which like all the other books mentioned is in increasing demand, is also of interest to physicians.

All this is a hopeful sign that *F. X. Mayr's* work, which can be such benefit to people today, will continue to find larger audiences.

---

* Now in its 38th edition.

May all the readers of this 30th edition learn something valuable from it and successfully experience *F. X. Mayr*'s proven path to recovery.

A-9082 Maria Wörth-Wörthersee,
August 1980   *Erich Rauch*, M.D.

Part I

Illness and Health — a New View

Boerhaave, Semmelweis, Mayr: Men ahead of their time

Boerhaave, the greatest physician of his day, died 200 years ago. During his lifetime he announced plans to bequeath the sum of his medical knowledge to his contemporaries for the benefit of both the sick and the well.

After his death, scientists from every corner of the earth gathered for the sale of his sealed work. Imagine their surprise, especially that of the wealthy Englishman who had bought it at such a high price, when they opened its pages only to find them blank except for the following couplet penned on the last page:

> "Keep the head cool and warm the feet,
> And carefully watch how much you eat!"

A joke? Hardly—rather, a golden rule for a healthy way of life, easy to understand and yet misunderstood by most. There is something peculiar about the truth: the simpler it is, the easier it is to disregard.

Less than a hundred years later, *Philipp Ignaz Semmelweis,* having discovered the cause of puerpural fever, spent the rest of his days in misery and ended up in an insane asylum! At that time almost half the mothers who had just given birth at a Viennese women's clinic were dying from puerpural fever. Frantic efforts to discover the cause of this horrible epidemic were in vain.

Semmelweis suspected that the physicians' hands, which went from performing autopsies to treating expectant mothers, were probably not completely clean. The doctors argued that they had always washed up before examinations, that their hands were therefore clean and could not possibly transmit any toxins. Anyone who thought otherwise was obviously crazy, a dreamer. They scorned *Semmelweis.*

But he went on to prove that the very hands that seemed so clean, were indeed contaminated. It was just such practices, he said, that were spreading unknown toxins from the dead to the living patients, and causing the death of countless young women. By establishing a very thorough method of handwashing, *Semmelweis* was able to stop the spread of infection. *Semmelweis*'s discovery marked a new age in hygiene, surgery and gynocology. He was hailed as the "savior of women" and a revolutionary in the field of medicine—but only after his death. During his lifetime he was ridiculed and opposed; his discovery was too novel, too simple and too important.

Dr. *Franz Xaver Mayr,* an Austrian contemporary, asserted the novel idea that the digestive systems of most people were not clean, no longer completely efficient and therefore unhealthy. Waste products deposited in the system caused it to be contaminated, often infected, and therefore a dangerous source of toxicity. This was undermining people's health and making them prematurely ill, old and unattractive.

Dr. *Mayr* insisted that everyone who was not completely well should thoroughly cleanse his intestines. But—just as Semmelweis before him, he meant something quite different than his contemporaries! He also held that digestive systems thought to be clean and healthy were, in fact, already more or less impaired and overrun with waste deposits.

How *Mayr* came to these conclusions is explained by his background:

Around the turn of the century, *Mayr* was a medical student working in a sanatorium where he treated people with intestinal problems. He wondered how he would know when he had reached the goal of his treatment, that is, wellness.

As he didn't have any reliable criteria for a healthy intestinal tract nor even for healthy people, he turned to the medical superintendent of the sanatorium, then to medical texts and finally to his teacher at the university with the questions:

1. How do we recognize good health in general and a healthy digestive system in particular?
2. What are the external signs of a healthy intestines? How are these reflected in the size, shape and condition of the abdomen? Can we tell by these signs, when the intestines are no longer healthy?

But nobody knew the answers.

The answer to these questions became a lifelong search for *Mayr.* Is a person who shows no signs of ill health, always completely well? Or is he only in a state of apparent health with illness lying secretly in wait? And is the digestive system we regard as normal, always really healthy, i.e. working efficiently and free of any deposits?

To answer this question he treated all his patients, regardless of whether they came to him with head, throat, lung, heart, stomach or abdominal complaints, as though they had digestive problems. Just as *Semmelweis* always had examining physicians wash their hands with embarrassing thoroughness, *Mayr* called for a thorough cleansing of all his patients' digestive organs, even those that seemed to be completely healthy. As a result, he came to the astonishing conclusion that:

1. even apparently healthy digestive systems are not completely healthy, in fact some have already suffered damage (deposits), and
2. by cleansing the digestive system and returning it to health, most other complaints, e.g. lungs, heart, stomach, etc., either abated or disappeared altogether.

After decades of research based on a unique series of examinations and treating thousands of patients, *Mayr* finally established the criteria for a healthy body, which he summarized in his "Diagnostics of Good Health".

Based on this, the following can be determined:

1. How far a person's state of health deviates from his optimal condition. (Damage to organs, preliminary stages of illness and states of illness previously unobserved are objectively ascertainable*.)
2. Whether a person's health has improved or deteriorated.
3. Which factors have a positive or negative influence on health.

With this set of diagnostics *Mayr* established the teaching or science of wellness, which had as its goal recognizing and maintaining the best possible state of health.

As medical science has always concerned itself intensely with disease, but rarely with health and healthy people, millions are spent every year on curing the sick or relieving them of specific symptoms. On the other hand, *very little of a serious nature is done to prevent*

---

* See previously unobserved signs of damage in illustrations 2 and 3.

*illness from occuring in the first place or to limit it to the expenditure of
vitality that is unavoidable with increasing age.* Without any diagnostics for good health, many danger signs cannot be recognized and
people cannot protect themselves in time. Since prevention is better
than a cure, Dr. *Mayr's* work on *maintaining wellness* was significant
as a basis for and complement to medical science, which till then
had been oriented towards *curing disease.*

Since being well or being sick — aside from genetic influences,
attack by dangerous pathogenic organisms or other drastic factors —
is mainly rooted in the way we live and eat, *basic good health, which
was Dr. Mayr's goal, cannot be purchased passivly, for instance simply
by taking pills. It unfolds gradually through the active participation of
the person seeking help, because this goal can never be reached without
struggling against bad habits. The decision therefore is a moral one!*

*Thus this path cannot be taken by those who are caught up in the
pursuit of pleasure, who have no self-discipline; nor by those who are
hampered by lack of understanding or a "know-it-all attitude".*

Like *Boerhaave* and *Semmelweis, Mayr* viewed illness and health in
a new light and, by pointing in a new direction, was therefore far
ahead of his time.

When and how illness begins

Illness is a drama in 10 acts: acts 1—3 take place totally unbe-
knownst; acts 4—6 unfold in the doctor's waiting room jammed
with patients; acts 7—9 in the hospital, and the last act on the
deathbed.

This can be confirmed from personal experience. One day you are
sick from some so-called "disease of civilization", e.g. rheumatism,
angina pectoris, stomach ulcers or colitis, hardening of the arteries,
high blood pressure, cancer etc., or you observe some of their symptoms, such as heartburn, a ravenous appetite, constipation, blood in
the stool, tension, fatigue, insomnia, headaches, backaches or stomach pains, loss of weight and the like, leading you naturally to
think that only one specific, immediate cause, such as catching a
chill, overexertion, or something lacking in your diet is solely responsible. Since you felt fine until now and had casually boasted
about never being sick a day in your life, you completely overlook

the fact that the cause which you are blaming for everything already represents the curtain rising on the 4th or 5th act. The previous acts have already been performed — without your knowledge.

It's later than you think!

Reads a sign in the waiting room of a Bavarian physician. How true.

It is an undeniable fact that most human beings are no longer healthy — in the fullest sense of the word —, but are at best in a state of apparent healthiness, artificially maintained.

"Diagnostics of Good Health" describes the preliminary stages of a decline in health so that someone in apparent good health can recognize the danger signs in time, prevent their occurence and initiate a recovery.

The question then arises: *when and how does this damage first occur?*

This is sometimes due to inherited organic weaknesses, predispositions and defects and sometimes to the habit of overloading the digestive system even in the first months of life, the reason being that most mothers believe only eating a lot will make a baby grow big and strong. They squeeze the contents of their breasts tirelessly into the mouths of their hapless babes; even the fully satisfied infant who has peacefully fallen asleep at the breast is awakened and encouraged to drink more. Openings in the nipples of baby bottles are too large, so that instead of drinking small digestible portions, children have to gulp down large amounts of milk just to keep up with the strong flow.

Mothers follow in the footsteps of grandmothers, those experts in child rearing. With the words "a spoonful for grandma, a spoonful for grandpa ..." the child who really doesn't feel like eating any more, is brought into line by gentle coersion and continues to be fed mercilessly. The next meal arrives before his stomach has finished digesting the last one. And little nibbles of this or that between meals assure that the digestive organs are working constantly.

A baby, tries vainly to defend itself by spitting up the overabundance of food. The saying "A baby that spits up is a healthy baby" is soon no longer applicable because vomiting and satiation reflexes don't function anymore. Instead, the baby's stomach gets sluggish and stretched out, the excess food ferments or decomposes in its intestines and leads to a qualitatively deficient diet despite the ample intake of food. To make up for this lack its appetite often increases. The child, poorly nourished by a maternal instinct to feed, overwhelmed by parental anxiety and a victim of old-fashioned ideas, now eats a lot and often — now he's "a good baby". This typical story proves that *a person is not born an overeater, but is raised to be one!*

However, the constant need to eat sometimes has the opposite effect: a psychological and physical aversion to eating. The result is a thin, pale child who slumps in his chair and is labeled a picky, nervous eater with no appetite. He already suffers from considerable digestive disturbances and is frequently the object of his relatives' concern and protracted treatment by doctors.

In both cases, no matter how different they may seem, the natural instinct, which should control the satisfaction of nutritional needs, is lost. Eating because it tastes good and as an end in itself, with either the quantity or a very selective quality being the determining factor — without any notion of the proper amount of food — replaces this natural instinct.

Anyone in this situation, who still thinks he is healthy, can actually only count on a semblance of good health and chronic digestive disturbances, which form the hidden beginnings of most illness.

The digestive system — roots of the human plant

The digestive system, a tube-shaped canal up to 27 feet long in adult human beings, begins with the lips of the mouth and ends at the anus. It includes the oral cavity, throat, esophagus, stomach, and the small and large intestines. Other glands are also part of it, such as the salivary glands in the mouth, the liver and gall bladder, the pancreas, as well as billions of mucous glands in the stomach and intestines (see ill. 1).

Normal digestion is achieved by the compatibility and cooperation of all these parts.

Digestion does not mean, as many think, the production of a stool, but rather:

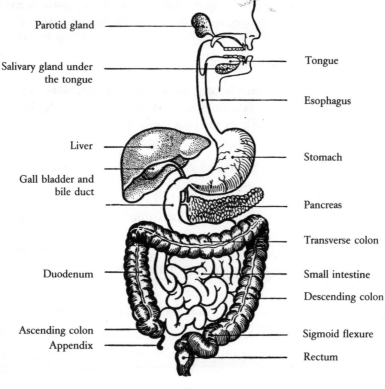

Parotid gland

Salivary gland under
the tongue

Liver

Gall bladder and
bile duct

Duodenum

Ascending colon
Appendix

Tongue

Esophagus

Stomach

Pancreas

Transverse colon

Small intestine
Descending colon

Sigmoid flexure

Rectum

Ill. 1
Human digestive system

1. *the correct mechanical, chemical and bacterial breakdown of nourishment, and its conversion into bodily substance and strength; and*
2. *eliminating unused waste products on time.* Opposing this normal process of digestion are the ordinary processes of fermentation and decay that cause disease (see p. 19).

Just as the small feeder roots of a plant absorb nourishment from the earth, producing branches, leaves and blossoms, countless intestinal villi take root in the chyme, absorbing food that has been broken down in the digestive system and supplying it to the bloodstream, which in turn carries it to all the areas that need it (the 33 billion cells of the body).

Besides the job of *nourishing the body,* the digestive system serves another basic function, which Dr. *Mayr* was the first to point out:

Purification of the blood

Like waste water from a factory, metabolic refuse released by every cell in the body has to be eliminated quickly and completely. To do this, the cell casts it off, so to speak, into the bloodstream, which immediately carries it to the excretory organs:

— The *lungs* exhale poisonous carbon dioxide and other gaseous waste products
— The *kidneys* excrete urine
— The *skin* eliminates waste products through cutaneous respiration (evaporation) and perspiration
— The *intestines* purify the blood of waste matter deposited in it and eliminates it in the stool (= blood purification by intestinal action).

For this reason the *stool* is made up of two components:

1. unused food particles (cellulose etc.);
2. waste products of intercellular metabolism that come from blood purification.

The *stool* created by a healthy digestive system should have the following properties:

Sausage-shaped, with rounded ends and a smooth surface encased in a mucousy sheath. It sinks in water because it has no gaseous impurities and has only a slight characteristic odor. It shouldn't smell either extremely foetid or extremely acidic, which are signs of intestinal putrefaction or intestinal fermentation. A healthy intestines evacuates the stool cleanly, which is why any noticable soiling of the anal region is an indication of damage to the intestinal tract. The huge amount of toilet paper we use these days is not a measure of civilization, but a deplorable sign of widespread chronic intestinal damage. Even animals such as dogs, cats, horses, goats, rabbits, deer, etc., as long as they are healthy, do not soil themselves when defecating. Veterinarians recognize the opposite as the sign of a diseased intestines. It is therefore unreasonable to assume that human beings, of all creatures, should be such a sorry exception.

Intestinal sluggishness leads to illness

Sluggish bowels have always been thought to mean sluggishness of the large intestine, and to be manifest by constipation. In fact, people thought sluggish bowels and constipation were one and the same thing.

Dr. *Mayr* was the first to point out that the small intestine (6—7 yards long!) can also function deficiently. Since the small intestine handles the most basic jobs of nutrition and blood purification, its impairment (action that is too slow or too rapid, "dysfunction", inflammation, etc.) is far more serious than that of the large intestine.

Whereas most pain, e.g. to sensory organs, the nerves, or the heart, registers almost immediately, unmistakably, even alarmingly, injury to the small intestine is an insideous process. Aside from the most acute pain, the person affected, usually notices very little or nothing at all. Symptoms like a feeling of fullness, flatulence, stabbing pains, abdominal pressure, or secondary symptoms like head congestion, shortness of breath, palpitations, unpleasant body odor, depression and so on are almost never blamed on the guilty small intestine. Moreover, bowel movements, even when there is serious damage to the small intestine, can sometimes be "like clockwork". But constipation and "sluggishness", even runny stools (process of decomposition!) or diarrhea are more often the case.

Thus, trying to evaluate the condition of the intestines from the stool alone is a disastrous, but unfortunately widespread error. The quality of the stool is by no means a reflection of the condition of the intestinal tract! Vast numbers of people, fooled by the regularity of their bowel movements, search vainly for the cause of their sufferings without knowing that it is their intestines which are responsible. They don't realize that regularity alone is not a sign of a healthy bowel (see p. 18), nor that sluggishness of the small intestine, as a functional disorder, is not detectable by x-ray. *Mayr*'s diagnostics first made this fact known to x-ray technicians.

The results of chronic damage to the intestines are:

1. Formation of toxins from decomposition

Just as butter gets rancid in a warm pantry, fruit salad begins to ferment, meat, sausage and fish go bad and become toxic, a sluggish intestines forms poisons because further transport and the mixture of food pulp with digestive juices that prevent perishability have been interferred with.

By-products of fermentation, such as various alcohols, including toxic fusel, are formed from sugar, bread, fruit, vegetables and dishes prepared with flour.

Highly toxic substances arising from decomposition such as indican, putrescine, neurine and cadaverine (ptomaine), which are so poisonous that only a small dose given by injection is enough to kill a laboratory animal, are formed from protein-rich foods like meat, fish and eggs.

These poisons are not completely eliminated in the stool, but remain partly in the bloodstream. If the amount of poison is great enough or if the liver, the body's detoxifying organ, is itself damaged, which is the case with sluggish bowels, alcoholism (cirrhosis) etc., the poisons can perforate the liver's barrier and swamp the organism.

As a result, *secondary symptoms* may appear:

A general run-down condition, loss of interest in work, moodiness, irritability, nervousness, bad breath and body odor, coated tongue, back pains and lumbago, sleep disturbances, headaches or congestion, chest pains, shortness of breath, angiospasms (with constantly cold hands and feet), dizziness, exhaustion upon waking, heavy sweating etc. What is known as neuro-dystonia, migraine headaches, diseases stemming from hypertension such as neuralgia, joint disease etc. are often only secondary symptoms caused by the intestines.

Many people know the source of these signs of poisoning, since they occur or intensify during occasional constipation. People who are often constipated suffer from these symptoms almost constantly.

The result of this "autointoxication" is damage to all the cells and organs of the body, with the senses, nerves, blood vessels and glands being particularly affected.

2. Occurence of abnormal bacterial flora (non-physiological colonization of bacteria)

Normal colonies of bacteria in human beings act as important allies in certain metabolic processes and in the fight against germs. Dense races of bacteria populate the surface of our mucous membranes both inside and outside the intestines. Normal intestinal bacteria can, among other things, destroy disease germs and parasites, improve overall health and manufacture useful substances like vitamins.

But in a large part of the central European population, this colonization process has been so disrupted that degenerative and parasitic bacterial forms proliferate, decomposing the contents of the intestines and producing toxins. If germ-killing antibiotics or other foreign bodies have not already damaged the bacterial flora, floral disruption and the spread of pathological microbes in the intestines occur where the intestines have been damaged, just as toads settle in and multiply where the ground is marshy.

3. Diseases of the digestive system

Sluggish bowels may eventually lead to gastritis and gastric ptosis, gastric and intestinal ulcers or various diseases of the small and large intestines accompanied by abdominal pains, flatulence, diarrhea or constipation; to liver, gallbladder and pancreatic dysfunctions; to hemorrhoids or finally even to intestinal cancer. The occurence of cancer in other organs may also have its primary cause in sluggish bowels because the bowels are the organism's major source of toxicity *(thus cleansing should also be done as a preventive measure!)*

4. Contamination of the body

If the intestines do not do their work of purifying the bloodstream effectively, the result may be a backup of metabolic wastes in the body, which causes a kind of "autointoxication". To get rid of these poisons and to protect vital organs, the body dumps this backed-up "garbage" into relatively less important tissues like adipose and connective tissue, tendons and muscles. But here too, pockets of chronic disease begin to develope over a period of time, especially if these deposits continue to build up. In its advanced stages, every organ of the body is affected.

Deposits of waste products and other residues produce:

In adipose and muscle tissue:	Adipose tissue and muscle rheumatism (gelosis)
On the vertebrae:	Spondylosis

In the joints:	Arthrosis, arthropathy
In internal organs:	Organic degeneration (e.g. of the heart, liver, kidneys, etc.)
In the arteries:	Hardening of the arteries, esp. the capillaries (early stages of angina pectoris, myocardial infarction)
In the gall bladder or kidneys:	Gall or kidney stones
On the skin:	Acne, rashes, pasty complexion, age spots, etc.

5. Malnutrition of all the cells in the body

Poorly nourished cells and organs are less efficient and less resistant: the skeletal muscles tire more quickly and do less work, the cardiac muscles are prone to heart disease, poorly nourished brain cells mean forgetfulness, poorly nourished testicular cells cause premature aging (as well as secondary symptoms).

6. Mental well-being of the entire person is eventually affected

As auto-intoxication spreads through the entire body, those parts of the organically-based nervous system which transmit spiritual processes to the body, also become affected. If this neuro-vegetative "organ of conveyance" is damaged by poisons, it is difficult for spiritual sensations to reach the brain centers that control physical consciousness. The following personality changes may take place: abandoning previous ambitions and ideals, shallowness, unkindness, increased egoism, materialism and ruthlessness. (Simply removing toxins from the body cannot turn a "bad" person into a "good" person; however, it can put him more in touch with his higher emotions, which would have a very positive effect on his total personality. This is why all world religions have practiced fasting since time immemorial [see p. 35].)

Inevitably, sluggish bowels are linked to imbalances in the brain as the seat of imagination and memory, not to mention changes in temperament, depression and irritability, as these processes are heavily influenced by any physical change. Slower thought processes, increased forgetfulness, melancholia, etc. need not always be attributed to daily preoccupations or even aging, but rather to metabolic poisoning of the brain.

Case history 1: Businesswoman, age 58, obese, bad eating habits, with an apparently healthy digestive system; disagreeable, ill-tempered, irritable, depressed, pessimistic, "my life has no meaning or joy"; unable to do a good job at work anymore. Forced to sell her failing business. Just before the last payment that would finalize the sale of the company, she went through Mayr inner body cleansing therapy. Her health returned to such a degree that, filled with new energy, zeal and *joie de vivre,* she revoked the sale and in a short time had her business in the red. Confident, friendly and happy again, this woman now seems younger and more active than she was 10 years ago!

Sluggish bowels lead to unattractiveness

1. Posture

As a result of his research into clearly identifiable signs of good health, *Dr. Mayr* established no less than 6 different types of abnormal posture, which he named after their characteristic features (see ill. 2b—g). They are not simply detractions from good looks, attributable to slovenliness or age, but constitute nature's emergency measures. Assuming no other infirmities or physical changes are present, for instance tumors, injuries, pregnancy, etc., abnormal posture is always a protective reaction to damaged digestive organs.

To inspect one's own posture, stand sideways in front of a mirror in a completely relaxed position. Any deviation from normal posture points to deeper causes.

A serious example of this condition is the *"duck" posture,* which is especially common in women (see ill. 2d). In this case the upper part of the body is thrust forward from the hips and then curves back over to counterbalance the buttocks, which sticks out in back. At every step the buttocks sways like a waddling duck.

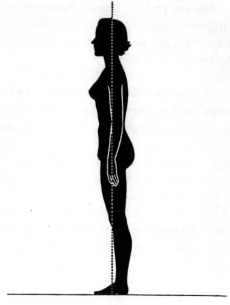

Ill. 2a
Normal posture

The duck stance, which is often the butt of jokes, is caused by chronic digestive damage (sluggish intestines). A healthy small intestine will not crowd any other organs when it occupies its natural place in the abdomen, but prolapsed intestinal loops, overloaded with half-digested food, put such pressure on neighboring organs, like the ovaries, uterus, vagina, urinary bladder and all their blood vessels, that the body assumes a posture of "making room" in an attempt to protect these sensitive organs.

One can see at a glance from each of the postures shown in ill. 2b-2g which disturbances or which illnesses each person will suffer from or will be strongly prone to. For instance, someone with "duck posture" will suffer from:

Digestive complaints, such as frequent constipation,
burping, heartburn, gas (result of sluggish intestines)
Gallbladder trouble (result of sluggish intestines)
Hemorrhoids (result of sluggish intestines)
Muscular rheumatism (sign of toxic deposits)

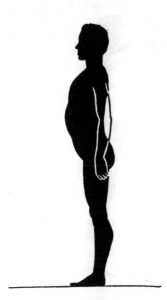 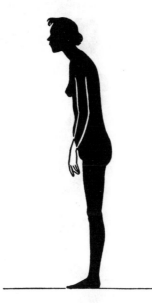

Ill. 2b
Abnormal posture: "Attention"
Due to chronic digestive damage (esp. to the epigastric region), the overstuffed stomach and intestines need more room. The thoracic section of the spine is bowed inward, especially in the case of muscular people, accompanied by increased arching of the chest cavity, elevation of the diaphram, and backward thrust of the lower part of the body with a drop in the pelvic floor.

Ill. 2c
Abnormal posture: Head start
This particularly affects people with poor musculature and tense abdominal walls. Chronic intestinal slackness increases the contents of the abdominal cavity and causes an enlargement of the abdomen. This stretches the spine, thrusting the upper part of the body forward, and causing the abdomen to protrude. In its extreme form, this posture is characterized by hunching over as though suffering from stomach cramps ("stomach ache posture").

Lower back pains (due to curvature of the spine) Menstrual disturbances, such as cramps, irregularity, difficulty in achieving sexual climax, and
Vaginal prolapse, predisposition to cystitis and urinary incontinence (due to constant pressure from the intestines on the pelvic region) and other complaints.

Case history 2: Housewife, age 52, duck posture since youth.
Parental admonishment and personal attempts to improve her posture, as well as years of posture exercises, were in vain. For the

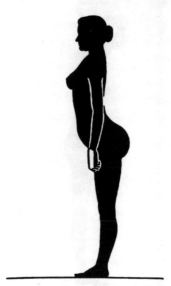 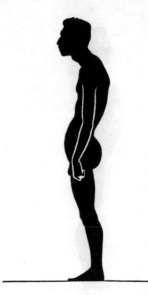

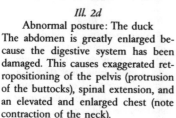

Ill. 2d
Abnormal posture: The duck
The abdomen is greatly enlarged because the digestive system has been
damaged. This causes exaggerated ret-
ropositioning of the pelvis (protrusion
of the buttocks), spinal extension, and
an elevated and enlarged chest (note
contraction of the neck).

Ill. 2e
Abnormal posture: Lazybones
Displacement of the center of gravity
is compensated for by the upper de-
flection of the spine (curvature) in people with poor musculature and glutted
intestines.

past 8 years she has been plagued by most of the characteristic complaints of the "duck lady". Patient currently receiving: series of injections, a wide range of pills, tablets, drops, suppositories, infusions,
radiation treatments, liniments, therapeutic packs, steam baths and
has had two stays at a health spa. Only after undergoing Mayr therapy for sluggish bowels did all her symptoms abate and her posture
become normal again. The clothes she had been wearing no longer
fit her. Use of drugs has become completely unnecessary.

Case history 3: Produce clerk, female, age 59, duck posture, thinks
she has a sound digestive system. Twice underwent surgery to correct urinary incontinence, but this was unsuccessful in the long run.
A sudden cough or wrong movement was enough — especially if
she was standing for long periods of time at the grocery store and

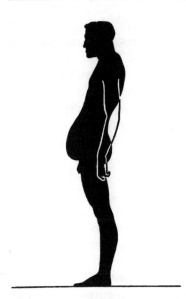

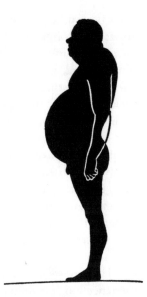

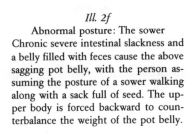

Ill. 2f
Abnormal posture: The sower
Chronic severe intestinal slackness and a belly filled with feces cause the above sagging pot belly, with the person assuming the posture of a sower walking along with a sack full of seed. The upper body is forced backward to counterbalance the weight of the pot belly.

Ill. 2g
Abnormal posture: The bass drum player
Is like a soldier carrying the big bass drum in front of him. The tremendous increase in the contents of the abdominal cavity is caused by a gas or feces-filled belly. Extreme upward and outward thrust of the chest (neck disappears, head stuck between the shoulders, see also ill. 3c), compensatory curvature of the thoracic region of the spine, with the lumbar section curved inward, are signs of a serious disorder of the digestive system.

particularly in winter — to cause urine to flow down her legs. The smell of the urine was occasionally so strong that customers and aquaintances noticed it. Tests revealed severe slackening of the small intestine, the weight of which was pressing on the urinary bladder. After 8 weeks in treatment her intestines had visibly tightened, her belly had shrunk and her posture had markedly improved. Existing high blood pressure, as well as the incontinence, disappeared completely. Since that time (6 years ago) the patient has remained dry — with annual therapy.

As can also be seen in illustrations 2b—2g, slackening of the intestines is accompanied by an increase in their contents, which in turn causes curvature of the spine to achieve balance. To prevent falling forward, anyone whose belly is filled with gas and feces has to assume the posture of the bass drum carrier (ill. 2g), with its concomitant curvature of the lumbar region of the spine. Finally, frequent painful irritation of the nerve roots, destruction of spinal segments, lower back pain, and all forms of sciatica and lumbago may occur as a result of overloading the spinal discs with excess body weight, especially the 4th and 5th lumbar vertebrae.

The most frequent treatment used these days to straighten vertebrae that have shifted or slipped out of position is chiropractic adjustment. Experience now shows that chiropractors have a much better success rate, and indeed it is sometimes the only way they can effect a long-term cure, if treatment is done in conjunction with Mayr Therapy, *which attacks the source of poor posture.* From my own experience too, a combination of the two natural forms of treatment produces excellent results (see also "typical cases", p. 55).

2. The skin*

A beautiful skin, and only healthy people have it, is pinkish, silky smooth, dense and tightly elastic. It clings firmly, covering the body like a perfectly fitted, unwrinkled pair of tights. It softens the irregularity of its foundation, creating the beautiful contours we admire in a healthy person.

A wide range of toxins, for instance the poisons produced by addiction, fatigue and infection, or certain medications, change the skin if their effects are strong enough, and leave their characteristic stamp. By far the worst of these toxins are the intestinal toxins. They produce such changes in the skin, mucous membranes, hair and nails that the degree of autointoxication can actually be measured:

In the first phase of toxicity, the puffy stage, the elasticity of skin fibres and framework decrease, so that its original tight structure gets looser and softer and looks as if it were "swollen". Thus, from a

---

* Details can be found in the supplementary publication "Cleansing the Blood and Other Bodily Fluids", which describes how the effects of poor blood chemistry and bodily fluids are reflected in the facial skin, and illustrates them with colored pictures.

healthy, oval face (see ill. 3a) with cheeks located near the zygomatic arch, securely attached and firm as apples, comes the moon-face (ill. 3b), which seems to be healthy, in fact overly-healthy, but which in reality already suggests a "state of deficient health". The cheeks form lower on the face and are so soft and flabby that they quiver like jelly at every shake of the head. Corresponding changes occur throughout the whole body. Healthy, well-formed, curvaceous arms and legs are no longer well-proportioned, and the beautiful curves of a healthy torso melt into unshapeliness.

In the second phase of toxicity, the flaccid stage, the loss of skin elasticity is even more pronounced. The cheeks drop markedly under their own weight. Lines form around the corners of the nose and mouth, "laugh lines" appear, as well as a double chin and rings on the neck (ill. 3c); the breasts, belly and rump sag, rings appear below the buttocks and the lower part of the body spreads out into a shapeless, blubbery mass.

In the third phase of toxicity, thinning of the skin, essential cutaneous components atrophy.

The skin is thinner, lacks tone and is so pliable that it sinks into the cavities of its foundation. Muscles and bones, especially the nose, chin and cheek bones, protrude and the figure becomes more angular. The eyes also look sunken (hollow-eyed).

In the first degree of this stage, the face is still unwrinkled, as in ill. 3d, but the thin skin has no tone and can easily be pulled away from its foundation.

In the second degree, the skin is even thinner and the face is deeply furrowed with wrinkles (ill. 3e).

In the third degree, the skin is only paper thin and looks almost creased in spots (ill. 3f).

The extent of damage to the organism from toxins can be diagnosed by these outward signs, and changes for the better or worse precisely noted. Skin elasticity (and thus any improvement or deterioration) can easily be judged by the fullness or flaccidity of the female breast by measuring the distance of the nipples from the upper sternum.

The relationship between colon toxicity and changes in cutaneous tissue, such as wrinkles, dewlaps, double chin or pendulous breasts, has been proven. Detoxification and improved functioning of the intestines cause these signs to retreat, unless they have already assumed irreparable proportions. The same also goes for many skin disorders like acne, boils, hives, eczema, ordinary blemishes, or for specific damage to hair and nails (splitting, brittleness, poor pigmentation). Since intestinal damage is the most frequent cause of impurities in the bloodstream, *improving the condition of the digestive system is the best and most natural means of improving one's looks.*

Aside from crisis-like reactions, positive changes in appearance gradually take place during Dr. *Mayr*'s intestinal cleansing treatment and become most pronounced a few months after therapy has been completed. Thus the results of a cure taken in summer often first show up as a "Christmas gift". The difference in photographs taken before and after therapy and then later on is frequently astonishing.

The connection between how a person looks and his state of health cannot be disputed:

Better health equals better looks!

Sluggishness of the bowels causes premature aging

Statistics show that the average expected lifespan is:

Table 1

During Roman times	30 years
Mid-17th century	35 years
Eighteenth century	36 years
Beginning of 19th century	40 years
End of the 19th century	45 years
1911	46.6 years
1920	55 years
1944	64 years
1954	68.2 years

This development is due to improved hygiene (successful control of epidemics and infectious diseases) and to the drop in infant mortality. Changes in nutrition, influenced by experiences in both world wars, have also increased life expectancy in the last few decades.

Compared with the past, people generally eat much less and it is of better quality. What served 3 in grandmother's cookbook would feed 5 or 6 today.

A well-balanced diet and more modest portions have also contributed to a longer lifespan. However, the hope for a happy old age, free from crippling and painful infirmities, really depends on controlling arteriosclerosis. This disease — resulting in high blood pressure, stroke, heart attack, physical and metal senescence — is a very frequent cause of pain, illness and death.

To forestall arteriosclerosis, one should be aware that the build-up of serum cholesterol and calcium in the arteries can begin even in childhood. Post-mortems on 300 American soldiers killed in the Korean War (average age 22!) showed that 77 % of them already had visible signs of hardening of the coronary blood vessels!

But the course of this insidious disease *can* be controlled. Its development ist hastened by foods rich in fat, cholesterol and sugar. For instance, in parts of China where rice is the dietary staple, people have almost no signs of hardening of the arteries, whereas the Eskimos, whose diet relies heavily on fat and meat, die from its effects at an average age of 40! Yeminite Jews, who eat no sugar at all, don't have any form of arteriosclerosis. However, those who emigrate from Israel and begin to eat sugar get hardening of the arteries, while those who remain faithful to Yeminite dietary laws are spared.

Furthermore, the process of hardening of the arteries is aggravated by sluggish intestines, which is the main cause of the build-up of contaminants (see p. 19). Cleansing and rejuvenating the digestive tract can reduce the level of sugar and chloresterol in the blood, which in turn combats arteriosclerosis.

Dr. *Mayr*'s proposal that everyone, regardless of age, cleanse his inner body from time to time would also help, besides being very important to the health of the individual and to the population as a whole.

Hormonal glands (pituitary, thyroid, gonads, adrenals) also largely determine a person's state of youthfulness or age; the ability of these glands to function properly is influenced by nutrition as well as by how much toxicity they contain. Any good cleansing will have a positive effect on the way they function, which leads in turn to a rejuvenation that can be seen and felt.

Professor *Kollath* stated that *"age is determined not by years, but by habits of living and eating; date of birth is inconsequential"*, to which Dr. *Mayr* added:

"It can be proven that toxins in the bowels make people ill, prematurely old and unattractive."

But an old folk saying puts it short and to the point:

"Death lurks in the intestines".

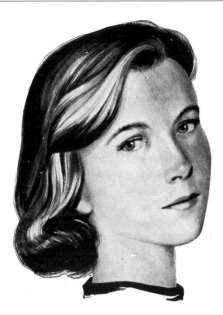

Ill. 3 a
Normal physiognomy
(see p. 29)

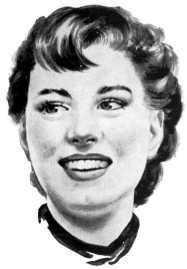

Ill. 3 b
Puffy stage
(see p. 29)

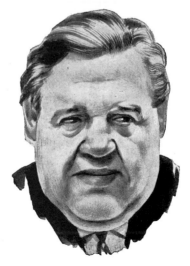

Ill. 3 c
Flaccid stage
(see p. 29)

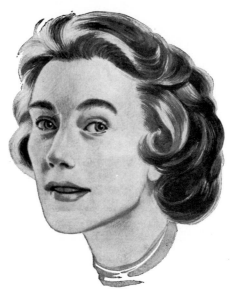

Ill. 3d
Thinning of the skin
1st degree
(see p. 29)

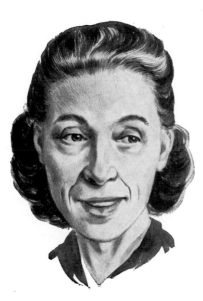

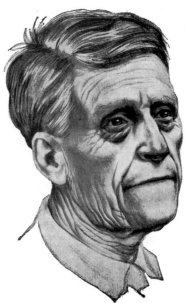

Ill. 3e
Thinning of the skin
2nd degree
(see p. 29)

Ill. 3f
Thinning of the skin
3rd degree
(see p. 29)

Part II

Recovery by the Mayr Plan

Health care

Medicine of the future will primarily be preventive medicine: medicine that does not rely merely on detecting early signs of existing diseases by using laboratory-oriented check-ups, but much more active preventive medicine, one which will train and counsel so-called „well people" about what positive actions they can take to maintain and improve their health. Its main focus will be a health-conscious reorientation towards ways of living and eating, such as natural psychosomatic training and therapy. People who have seriously fasted or undergone inner body cleansing know from their own experience what a pleasant effect this can have on both body and mind; they know the importance of intestinal, blood, fluids and tissue cleansing; and they know how necessary and valuable detoxifying and decontaminating the system is for modern man, even as a preventive tool.

We take for granted that we have to have our automobile serviced every few thousand miles to prevent things from going wrong with it. Neither money, time nor energy is spared for this purpose. Yet we have almost no idea that, to maintain our health, there are essential things that we can and should actively do! The usual attitude toward health is incredibly passive today because we get either insufficient or false information. Like naive children, we take good health for granted. A sense of responsibility for one's own health often arises only when wracking symptoms of illness appear. Life insurance companies have yet to include active health care in their educational and claims programs, although active prevention is the only real way to reduce the explosion of costs in public health. *"An ounce of prevention is worth of pound of cure"* is an old saying, but truer today than ever.
Yet the simple phrase
Your health-the unknown creature
still typifies people from affluent societies who, for all their thou-

sands of complaints, are completely uninformed about active prevention and health care.

There are numerous reasons for this ignorance. One of them is
that the teachings of *F. X. Mayr* are largely unknown. *Paracelsus* was
right when he demanded that the sick be recognized by the external
signs of their sickness, their "signatures", just as fools were identified
by their bells. *F. X. Mayr* was able to describe the visible signatures
of numerous internal diseases by using diagnostics and he showed
how they could be recognized and treated in their early stages. People whose eyes have been opened by *Mayr*'s diagnostics will meet at
every step so-called healthy people who are in fact just half-sick people against a backdrop of sick people: the base drum players, the
sowers, the duck ladies, the wizened-up, those bursting their buttons
with pot bellies, and many others, all mainly characterized by poor
nutrition and poor digestion.

You only have to go the beach once and critically observe the
figures, bellies and skin conditions of the bathers to see that at least
every other one demonstrates characteristic features of poor nutrition and digestion. Yet very few of them are aware of their condition
and most act like they have a monopoly on good health, burning the
candle at both ends, drinking too much coffee, snacking constantly,
taking medicines and drugs, until one day *"it's later than you
think"!*

We have also observed the shapes of the bellies of patients who
are sent to health resorts (usually paid for by the state or social secu-
rity) and can see that the majority of these are also primarily cases of
poor nutrition and digestion.

Yet these same patients (if the spa staff is not versed in Dr. *Mayr*'s
diagnostics) will be fed an amazingly rich diet; and many will even
takes seconds of desserts, coffee, and drinks since swimming and
lying around make one hungry and thirsty. This only impairs the
process of detoxification and elimination of metabolic wastes begun
by therapy and intensifies *the most common disease of people living in
a civilized, affluent society: damage to the alimentary/digestive/meta-
bolic systems.* Sometimes it isn't long before the patient has to go
through therapy again or start using expensive drugs.

Dr. *Mayr*'s diagnostics prove objectively that for modern civilized
man, a "health service", involving a course of fasting, intestinal
cleansing and detoxification, done as early as possible, is absolutely

appropriate and necessary. And moreover, that the early stages of damage and preliminary disease processes can usually be reversed by taking such measures. And last but not least, that the seeds of preventable illnesses still germinating in the body can to a large extent be halted. *Thus Mayr's treatment method is a highly effective, active health care program, which can be very beneficial to modern man.*

We aren't saying anything new by recommending this kind of preventive medicine. We are only repeating the centuries-old message of all civilized religions concerning temporary or partial fasting. *F. X. Mayr* merely took this ancient knowledge and made it diagnostically verifiable and easy to use by adapting it to contemporary lifestyles.

Therapeutic fasting

Our knowledge of the cleansing and rejuvenating powers of fasting is ancient. By fasting we mean the temporary, voluntary limitation or complete suspension of food intake. It was and is a vital part of religious ritual for countless peoples. No major religious system exists which does not recommend, even order, that its followers cleanse their bodies and souls with annual fasting in order to release them from impurities and illness and to elevate them to the recognition and attainment of higher ends. Even early schools of philosophy (Pythagoreans, Stoics, Epicureans, etc.) used fasting to attain physical fitness and thus approach the perception of truth and rigorous self-control. The great physicians of antiquity, such as *Hippocrates* and others, whose intuitive knowledge we still admire, often made use of fasting. As modern medicine increasingly relies on this most natural of remedies, it is only following a practice that is probably as old as the human race itself.

Fasting allows the digestive system to rest and recuperate; it cleans and detoxifies the organism of metabolic wastes and mobilizes its powers of healing to combat disease processes.

Fasting has proven effective against a large number of illnesses: digestive, metabolic and glandular illnesses; obesity, heart and circulatory problems; many respiratory diseases, illnesses relating to the female kidneys, bladder and abdomen; various skin conditions and allergic reactions; all types of fevers, as well as certain nervous and mental disturbances.

Moreover, when used early enough, fasting is the preventive method par excellence for stopping the outbreak of numerous illnesses, for improving overall health and increasing energy.

Fasting owes its intense curative powers to such descriptions as "operation without a knife" and "the royal path to recovery".

Fasting is much different than hunger.

Hunger is defined as a lack of sufficient nutrition to the point where the body suffers. This can occur:

1. internationally, by going on a hunger strike or doing "hunger therapy";
2. unintentionally, as a result of lack of food, famine, disasters;
3. by a major imbalance in the digestive system, whereby the cells of the body are starved despite sufficient food intake.

Fasting, on the other hand, is a completely voluntary limitation of or abstinence from food in order to improve overall health. Such a cessation means a reasonable and beneficial rest and detoxification of the organism rather than any damaging loss of food supply. Whereas people who are hungry become more and more unhappy, especially if hunger is accompanied by a threat of starvation (for example, miners caught in a cave-in), the condition of those who fast appreciably improves. The entire organism becomes healthy again, any number of disturbances and complaints are relieved and there is a positive feeling of cleanness, a harmony between the inner and outer self. Fasting, the royal path to recovery, is backed by thousands of years of tradition and proven results and its great healing effects can only be disputed by the uninformed.

When Dr. *Mayr* and his patients first fasted, he was so impressed with the favorable results that he devoted the rest of his life to this method of healing. Various forms and levels of treatment came out of his experiences:

1. Mayr's tea fast

This is a strict form of fasting in which only weak herbal tea (with perhaps a little honey and lemon), water, mineral water, or clear vegetable broth is taken for either several days, for 1, 2, or 3 weeks, or even longer in special cases. Such a fast should be done under medical supervision, ideally at a sanatorium. It is also helpful not to think about work-related problems, to lay aside worries and cares and to place oneself in an atmosphere and climate that promote healing: quietness, good air, natural, undisturbed surroundings, as well as interaction with other people who are doing the same fast. The liberating experience of inner cleansing creates relaxed and positive personal relationships among its participants:

Fasting makes one freer and happier!

At a sanatorium there won't be any tiresome interferences from tactless or thoughtless friends. These types often try unconsciously to thwart the cure, either because they cannot imagine not eating or because they are jealous or feel guilty because they themselves should have fasted but were too fainthearted or weak-willed.

Mayr's tea fast differs from other therapeutic fasts in the following aspects:

1. The physician directing the cure is thoroughly versed in *Mayr*'s diagnostics, so that he gets a complete picture of the patient's general state of health, the degree of contamination and toxicity and the extent of fasting the patient needs.
2. The intensity and length of treatment can be determined and regulated for the individual by using objective measurable standards.
3. Criteria for determining the best post-treatment diet for a given patient *(important for long term success).*
4. The entire digestive system is cleansed in the natural direction, from the oral cavity downwards, by drinking a saline solution (see section on "Cleansing", p. 47), instead of partial cleansing in the opposite direction, from the anus upwards, by using enemas and colonics.
5. Manual abdominal treatment (MAT), performed by a physician, is a vital personal help toward a rapid return to good health (see section on "Training", p. 49).

The transition from tea fasting to a hard roll and milk diet and later to a modified elimination diet, with its special training in eating and chewing, exemplifies Dr. *Mayr*'s primary claim:

"Rather than teaching people how to fast, we need to teach them how to eat properly."

The normal length of time for complete *Mayr* therapy in a sanatorium is usually about 4 weeks — 3 weeks for an abbreviated treatment. Depending on the diagnosis, the course usually, though not always, goes from *Mayr*'s tea fast to a hard roll and milk diet and finally to a more managable type of diet plan.

2. Maintenance and cleansing therapy with a hard roll and milk diet (Mayr's milk fast)

Whereas the tea fast is only available to a limited number of people, namely sanatorium guests, practically anyone can go on one of the many milk fasts, including modified elimination therapy. The credit for this goes to Dr. *Mayr*, who made basically the same type of treatment as fasting accessible to people employed full-time, in the form of the milk fast or one of its modified versions:

"Fast without fasting".

Undergoing a mild form of treatment is quite easy for most people while still on the job. But this always requires medical supervision and manual abdominal treatment (MAT).

In addition, the milk fast also

a) teaches proper eating

Proper nourishment depends on eating correctly, which means always taking small bites, chewing them thoroughly and liquifying them quickly by means of a conscious, intense insalivation (this takes concentration). But almost nobody does this these days. Just as the muscles of the arm keep getting stronger and more efficient by throwing a javelin, atrophied salivary glands are strengthened by this type of eating therapy; they re-learn how to produce saliva of an ideal quality and quantity to digest a given food; they are able to thoroughly disinfect and clean the oral cavity after eating by rinsing it in thin saliva. Eating correctly also produces better teeth cleaning and improved circulation in the gums and roots of the teeth (massage effect from chewing), thus reducing the chance of gingivitis and loss of teeth. Some digestive functions can be performed more completely when eating is done correctly and this *lays the groundwork for recovery of the rest of the digestive tract.*

This is where *Mayr* therapy comes in. A person has to start over again from the beginning. He has to learn how to chew and insalivate and practice this regularly. And if he really works at it he can learn this art of eating so well it would take almost a lifetime to unlearn it.

Since no other method of fasting and no nutritional system, be it *Bircher-Benner, Jackson, Hauser, Waerland* or even more recently that of *Kollath* and others, teaches this prerequisite of proper nutrition, or does it only approximately as well as *Mayr* therapy, the latter when correctly done is, for this reason alone superior. It eliminates a primary source of bad nutrition and its resulting ailments.

b) makes use of a food that contains all the basic nutritional elements in a balance and is considered the classic decontaminant: milk.

It nourishes; it eases, intensifies and speeds up decontamination of the body; it reduces a crisis reaction or prevents it from occuring during cleansing treatment (details in later chapter).

c) provides an extremely long period of satiation at least twice a day to avoid any "feeling of hunger" or the fear of it.

d) is tailored as much as possible to individual needs, for instance as a transition to other maintenance diets.

e) Lengthof therapy is variable, depending on the patients's condition, the effectiveness of treatment, and or the physician's determination.

Each type of *Mayr* therapy, be it tea fast, milk fast or some other modified diet (see p. 51), is based on three principles:
A) respite, B) cleansing and C) training.

A) Respite

The idea of respite is derived from nature. A wild animal that is sick takes a rest so that it can concentrate all its energies on getting well again. It finds a protected place and lies down, instinctively taking no food or only very specific foods until it has recovered. Medical science has also used this principle since time immemorial: the mentally ill have to "convalesce", those with fever take to their beds, a broken arm is put in a sling, a broken leg in a cast.

Dr. *Mayr* allows the digestive organs to convalesce by fasting or by using the best possible mild diet.

Milk

Milk contains an unrivaled abundance of all the basic caloric carriers and vital substances in a harmonious balance: amino and fatty acids, vitamins, enzymes and minerals (including trace elements). It has antibiotic properties, is a decontaminant, our most important carrier of vital substances, a unique, secret "elixir of life", and rightly called the "queen of foods".

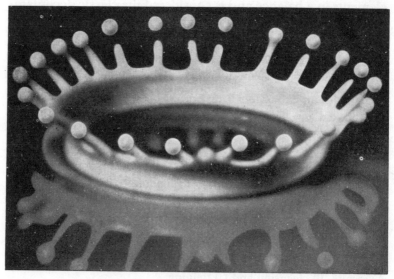

Ill. 4
A drop of milk — nature's miracle (enlarged photograph)

Table 2

Average composition of milk:

protein	3.5 %	potassium	0.160%
fat & lipoids	3.5 %	calcium	0.125%
lactose	4.8 %	magnesium	0.125%
water	87.5 %	iron	0.010%
total minerals	0.7 %	chlorine	0.106%
sodium chloride	0.157%	phosphorous	0.90%
	sodium	0.051%	

Average vitamin content in 1 litre of milk:

Vitamin A	0.6—2 mg	Choline		150 mg
Vitamin B1	0.4 mg	Vitamin C	5—	30 mg
Vitamin B2	1.6—2.5 mg	Vitamin D	0.002	mg
Niacin	1 mg	Vitamin E	0.6	mg
Pantothenic acid	2.8—4.5 mg	Vitamin F	1050—1750 mg
Vitamin B4	1—3 mg	Vitamin K	0.32	mg
Vitamin B12		2—3 micrograms

The biological value of milk can be shown by the growth of young animals, whose weight doubles or triples in a short period of time.

The best milk is fresh from the cow, followed by raw milk (grade A milk), then infant formula which, has only been warmed in hot water, rather than scalded. Changes already begin to take place in the protein or in the milk itself when it is heated above 45° C. Malted coffee (coffee made from an infusion of barley malt) added to milk, yoghurt from a health food store, or a good grade of sour milk can also be used.

Milk should not be thought of as a drink that is gulped down to quell one's thirst, but rather a liquid food to be *taken only in the smallest portions,* and like an infant only when needed, then thoroughly mixed with saliva. *Milk should be "eaten", not drunk.* To achieve this, Dr. *Mayr* suggests taking with it a good, chewy.

Hard roll

that promotes the production of saliva.

The consistency of the roll is critical to the success of the treatment. Only the right type of roll will increase the efficiency of the saliva glands, produce a stronger flow of saliva and at the same time train one to chew properly.

Ideally, rolls should be purchased fresh every day and spread out on wax paper or a towel to air dry. Depending on the weather, they will reach the desired consistency in two to four days: dry enough to be cut, sturdily elsatic, i.e. they can still be pressed in a little, but noticably harder than fresh hard rolls, though nowhere nearly as hard as rolls dried for bread crumbs.

It is absolutely necessary to be sure there is a sufficient backlog of rolls on hand and to check their condition before each meal so that just the right stale roll is used.

If the rolls remain too moist or too soft, the drying process can be accelerated by cutting them up and spreading out the pieces.

Rolls that are too soft or fresh don't have the absorbent properties of these "therapeutic" rolls, so they can't be sufficiently chewed and insalivated. They are poorly utilized by the body and don't satisfy as long; they can also cause abdominal distention and insufficient respite. This jeopardizes the entire treatment. Note: Rolls won't dry out in a steamy kitchen or in containers (breadbox, plastic bags, drawers).

Rolls that are bone dry and therefore too hard (rolls ready to be made into breadcrumbs, zwieback and toasted rolls) are also unsuitable. They are not absorbent enough, nor do they excite or maintain sufficient, flow of saliva; however, they are, relatively speaking, better than rolls that are too soft. They can also damage bad teeth. Note: Gas pains during therapy often means the wrong rolls or the wrong foods are being eaten.

Many health food practitioners think they cannot use *Mayr* therapy because these rolls have lost their food value through processing. Still others use whole wheat rolls instead. But they hevan't fully grasped the *Mayr* method; they are only thinking about vitamin intake and are forgetting that vitamins can't work if they are destroyed in an unhealthy digestive system. Taking vitamins is not the same as providing the cells of the body with vitamins, since their utilization is dependent on the health of the intestines. As most people in civilized societies do not have very healthy intestines, the best thing we can do to see that the body is supplied with vitamins is to make the intestines healthier by letting them go through a period of respite, cleansing and regeneration. Only then can a modest (!) rather than excessive amount of vital substances be available to the body in the form of natural foods. But not before!

Whole grain rolls eaten during the period of respite prevent the intestines from resting because of their high content of cellulose, which is indigestible. The rolls prescribed for the treatment, however, let the intestines rest as completely as they should.

Eating method

Just before you plan to eat it, cut a roll into thin slices. Put a small piece in your mouth and chew it well until saliva is produced (training the salivary glands). The bread and saliva will begin to form a watery paste with a slightly sweetish taste. Sweet because the starch in the bread is being converted into sugar by saliva enzymes. Now sip a small spoonful of milk, or better yet suck it from the spoon with lips almost pressed together. This sucking action creates a vacuum in the oral cavity and helps drain the salivary glands. (A baby at its mother's breast uses this type of sucking to insalivate each drink of milk!) Now mix the entire contents of your mouth — bread, saliva and milk — by more chewing and by using your tongue. This should taste good and the pleasure be savored. (Practice!). The milk is already starting to be vigorously digested in the oral cavity, which is essential to the success of the treatment. Now you can swallow the mixture. Repeat this process *until hunger is satisfied. Any amount may be eaten.*

This very specific way of eating is basic to the success of the *Mayr* treatment program:
1. Take small bites.
2. Chew and insalivate until the roll is liquified and a slightly sweet taste occurs.
3. Add a teaspoon of milk (never a mouthful!).
4. Mix well in the mouth and then swallow.
5. Eat only until satisfied. Don't eat what's left of either the bread or the milk! Take the milk by teaspoonsful with the bread mixture or not at all no exceptions!

Something worth having is worth working for. Here too, recuperation requires a cooperative attitude, honest effort, and following these steps thoroughly, consistently and with concentration, even though they may seem unimportant. This is *decisive.* After all, success is the goal! Treatment shouldn't even be started if this method of eating cannot be carried out. It must either be done right or not at all. Food well chewed is food half digested.

The tea

Two or three cups of herbal tea (linden blossom, fennel, yarrow, anserine, lemon balm, sage, etc.) with no more than a teaspoon of genuine bee honey (has trace elements) and a little lemon or orange juice (vitamin C) should be taken by spoonfuls(!) each evening.

It's best to buy herbal teas in a health food store, herb shop or naturopathic pharmacy where they are usually freshest.

Method: Pour boiling water over a pinch (the amount that can easily be picked up with three fingers) of tea, steep for only 1—2 minutes and then strain.

What to do if hungry or thirsty

If this treatment is followed exactly, you will feel satisfied longer than with normal eating. Any feeling of hunger between meals only occurs because eating was done incorrectly, too fast or otherwise carelessly, or because rolls were eaten that were probably too fresh. Always have something to drink when you are thirsty or when you eat.

Liquid diet: In general, liquids should be taken as often as possible during the day. Water, weak herbal tea or slightly carbonated mineral water are allowed. Drinks shouldn't be either too hot or too cold and should be swallowed in small amounts. Frequent intake of liquids greatly reinforces inner cleansing. If not contraindicated, 2 to 3 liters of liquid should be drunk every day if possible. If a feeling of hunger persists despite drinking warm tea, a bit of stale roll can be eaten between specified mealtimes, but always according to the method described. This feeling will disappear as health returns.

General care

Unless a person's health has been so impaired that treatment has to proceed in a sanatorium, it can be done by most people at home or on the job. This applies to those who do manual labor as well as to those who sit at a desk. Practically all types of professions lend themselves to parallel treatment — from butchers, mechanics, bakers, farmers, housewives, tailors, to judges, politicians and university professors. The only perequisite* is examination by a physician schooled in Dr. *Mayr*'s diagnostics and therapy. He will decide whether a person is best treated as an inpatient or outpatient. The advantage of

---

* Special training is also necessary for doctors who direct these cures. They must first undergo therapy themselves, because only with this personal experience can they completely grasp the total physical-spiritual event.

undergoing this very effective form of therapy as an outpatient, is that an individual need not even interrupt his work schedule. The obvious disadvantage is that *Mayr therapy should never be done without a Mayr physician.* It is easy to understand that such a fundamental therapy, such a drastic "general overhaul" of the entire organism, has to be directed and supervised by someone with experience. The type and length of treatment must be adapted to the demands of the patient and his responses. The diet has to be altered at just the right time, manual abdominal treatment (MAT) has to be done, and a proper transition to a modified diet and finally to healthier nutrition must be made. It is those things which determine to a large extent the success of the treatment.

Very often, coping with one's job seems to become less stressful even while treatment is in progress.

Bed rest is only prescribed in exceptional cases.

But as a general principle, quietness and rest are required. A few minutes to a half hour of rest before eating, short periods of relaxation when the opportunity presents itself and *retiring early on a regular basis* (being asleep before midnight) are *absolute requirements.* Watching TV every night oppresses the autonomic nervous system, interferes with deep sleep and therefore the regeneration of the organism. TV should not be watched during treatment! Any degree of tiredness, baths that are too hot, saunas* and steambaths* may precipitate a crisis and should therefore be avoided. There are also patients who need to take the opportunity of therapy to organize their everyday lives so that they are calmer, quieter and more balanced (harmony = husbanding strength). Confused thinking and behavior, burning the candle at both ends, constant hurrying and other stress factors should be avoided as much as possible once treatment has begun. (See p. 79 to p. 81 for the vital interaction between emotional and neurological factors.)

B) Cleansing

A report from Karlsbad, the world famous spa for digestive problems, relates: "I was sitting peacefully on my little bench in the woods, reading the newspaper, when suddenly somebody raced by,

---

* Normally very useful, but not during treatment.

tore the newspaper from my hands and disappeared. "Hey you", I yelled, "that's today's paper!" To which the voice responded, "Yes, but I can't wait for tomorrow's!"

Epsom (or Karlsbad) salts, taken every morning in a concentration equal to that of the blood, are also used in *Mayr* therapy for cleansing*. The advantage of this solution is that, unlike laxatives, it does not stimulate the intestinal mucous membranes. The salt water runs through the stomach and intestinal tract in the natural direction, gradually scaling bits of old, decomposed excrement and food from its walls and then flows out again. These deposits can settle for years in the recesses and folds of the 7—8 metres of intestinal tract, often bound up with the intestinal mucous membranes. They can be unbelievably poisonous. The effect and the amount of dissolved "slag" set in motion sometimes causes dramatic cleansing results (see above report). A diarrhea-like, liquid evacuation only occurs when intestinally-stimulating toxins have been dissolved. If these toxins are eliminated with the stool, the mucous membranes of the anus often get swollen and red and feel sore. Constipation can also occur and sometimes be slow to disappear if the toxins released have an immobilizing effect on the intestines. Loose or normal stools are also possible. But bowel movements usually become regular again after the first wave of toxins has been eliminated. Becoming regular again quickly, improved detoxification and a particularly *mild reaction can be achieved by drinking plenty of water, pure herbal tea or non-carbonated mineral water.* Unless otherwise indicated by the doctor, a daily total of 2—3 liters should be drunk at frequent intervals.

Even the most skeptical will be convinced by the results and therefore the necessity of cleansing therapy: a stool that comes only from eating milk and rolls is golden yellow and has almost no odor, not unlike a nursing infant's stool. Any other color and/or a bad smell indicate that incompletely digested, harmful residues are being eliminated.

These pollutants usually break up at the beginning of treatment, more often than not in the first few weeks. Unbelievable amounts of foul-smelling masses of stool, ranging in color from black, brown, and grey to white or green can be passed. Occasionally hard blocks

---

* 1 level teaspoon Epsom salts or Magnesium sulfuricum to ¼ liter lukewarm water. Wait to eat breakfast for at least half an hour.

of excrement as large as apples, skins, seed husks and other such characteristic meal residues from months past show up.* This process of dissolving can make the areas where these residues were attached sore. If bowel movements do not happen immediately in voluminous amounts, then they usually occur gradually, with less intensive coloration and less odor over a longer period of time. But even in the latter case, the appearance of consistently light yellow, odorless stools should result.

The entire body, including the blood, is also cleansed along with the intestines. Although cleansing mostly occurs in the intestines, all the areas and organs of secretion are involved: the kidneys (dark, cloudy, foul-smelling, "caustic" urine), the skin (sweating, body odor) and the mucous membranes, e.g. in the mouth and bronchial tubes (bad breath or unpleasant taste in the mouth, coated tongue), and for women the vaginal mucous membranes (vaginal discharge).

The longer and more intensely the body has had to endure this contamination, the longer it will take to thoroughly cleanse it. Thus when one of Father *Kneipp*'s patients in her so-called golden years became impatient after only a short time in treatment, he answered her pointedly: "You can't clean up such an old house in one day!"

C) Training

Nobody's intestines are damaged equally in all places. Slack, enfeebled sections and hypertonic sections that are overworked or pinched and spastic, alternate with normally-functioning parts. This is why training the intestines, i.e. returning them to normal activity, can never be done with chemical laxatives or foods that stimulate and stress (stewed plums, figs, sauerkraut, multi-grain dishes, kruska and the like). All of these stir up the entire intestines, which only further excites the already hypertonic, irritated and spastic portions, thus compounding the damage. The positive initial reaction of people who try to train their intestinal tract with mountains of linseed, fruit, grains etc., usually according to some health food advocate's "widely accepted recipes", quickly wanes. Here too, as with chemical laxatives, the quantity of live foods has to be increased gradually or

---

*Reports have recently come in about eliminating drug capsules that had been taken weeks before.

the inflammation of the intestines will spread. Unfortunately, the
damage some of these people do "schooling their intestines" may not
show up for years.

Dr. *Mayr*, on the other hand, uses an elaborate abdominal massage, called "manual abdominal treatment" (MAT). By applying vary-
ing degrees of mild pressure on the abdomen, a trained physician
can assess the present condition of various parts of the intestines and
can treat them accordingly.

MAT increases and decreases in rhythmic response to internal abdominal pressure, with the following results:

1. *Specific (characteristic to the species) intestinal activity is increased.*
   Resorption of nutrients into the blood stream becomes more intense, thus promoting elimination of waste products from the
   body into the intestines. After being treated for only a short time,
   the abdomen becomes measurably tauter, the diaphram drops,
   and the contents of the ascending colon become mostly liquid.

2. *Circulation in the abdominal cavity improves.* Blood and lymph
   fluids which have become dammed up at affected and inflamed
   sites are absorbed into the circulatory system and replaced by
   oxygen-rich blood or fresh lymph. Consequently, inflammation
   recedes quickly, leaving the patient free of pain caused by pressure. The sucking and pumping action of MAT supplies more
   blood to all the abdominal organs; during MAT this part of the
   body becomes warmer.

3. *The digestive glands make a steady recovery,* due to improved circulation and intestinal activity; for example, an enlarged liver gets
   rapidly smaller; the liver and gall bladder both become less sensitive to pressure.

4. *The blood is cleansed* because metabolic wastes are emptied more
   efficiently into the intestines, which are now working intensively.
   This is reflected in the tightening of facial skin. Wrinkles soften a
   little, producing a brighter expression and the complexion looks
   fresher and rosier. Cleansing the blood and stimulating circulation tones the heart muscles; this can be verified before and after
   each treatment through percussion and auscultation.

Dr. *Mayr's* MAT follows natural patterns. In a healthy organism,
the diaphram rises and falls rhythmically from abdominal breathing,
carrying out a natural "intestinal treatment", i.e. normal breathing in

healthy people acts like the motor for intestinal activity and abdominal circulation. However, if the digestive system is unhealthy, for instance from gastritis, inflammation of the small intestine, or an enlarged liver, normal breathing can't be tolerated; damaged organs need rest and relaxation in order to recover. Nature immediately compensates by a reflex reduction, or even blocking of abdominal breathing. Any teacher of respiratory exercises knows that very few people breathe correctly; their abdominal breathing is shallow, depending on how much damage has been done to the digestive system, and has been replaced by an irrational thoracic breathing. (The large number of people who breathe this way shows that there has been a tremendous increase in damage to the digestive system.) Moreover, the chest arches out and stiffens to protect unhealthy organs. A hump on the thorax, sensible to the trained eye and hand, appears in a spot that corresponds to the location of damage in the abdomen (e.g. liver, gall bladder, duodenal hump etc.*).

These changes, together with shallow breathing, prevent the alveoli, which carry out the exchange of gases during breathing, from emptying sufficiently (deflating). Thus, *the aeration of the lungs of people whose digestion is affected is always restricted.* They cannot completely exhale carbon dioxide (nor other gaseous products of metabolism that ought to be eliminated with it), so air remaining in the lungs keeps increasing. In the end this causes the blood to be overloaded with carbon dioxide, a slow form of autointoxication, which Dr. *Mayr* has shown us how to recognize and effectively counteract. Dr. *Mayr* has described MAT as artificial abdominal breathing. This very effective treatment also belongs only in the hands of a trained physician.

3. Maintenance and cleansing programs using a modified diet plan

People who cannot tolerate milk, even combined with barley-malt coffee or herbal tea, can substitute cottage cheese, gruel or mush made from wheat, oats, barley or rice.

---

* Details can be found in *Mayr*'s other books. Likewise *Schmiedecker: Liver Humps* (Med. Klin. 1958, 19). Practical experience with these diagnostic features is a prerequisite for proper intestinal treatment, since these changes, which occur in some form or another in almost everyone, have to be reversed.

Cream of wheat soup: Mix together 2 tbsp. whole wheat flour with 1 cup of cold water, bring to boil and boil 3 minutes, put through fine strainer, season with sea salt; use as substitute for milk with prescribed roll.

Oatmeal: Mix together 2 tsp. fine rolled oats or oat paste with cold water (the amount of water depends on desired thickness or thinness of the mush), bring to boil and boil 3 minutes; milk may be added or the yolk of 1 egg; spice with sea salt and soy sauce, if desired, and substitute for milk with prescribed roll.

Butter or a good margarine, honey, cottage cheese, or cream cheese can be used as a spread for the roll; soft boiled egg, may be used as a side dish; tender, steamed vegetables, fried potatoes, perhaps even braised veal or poached fish may also be used, but only on the advice of a physician. *Modified elimination therapy* is a very gently active treatment program, for which the *modified elimination diet* has been specially developed. Slight variations of the treatment also produce impressive results when they are tailored to an individual patient. The physician will find the best therapy by using Dr. *Mayr's* diagnostics.

The treatment

1. Introduction

The length and course of therapy depends on the patient's condition, his vitality and his healing quality, as well as on how closely he sticks to the program. Most people find the whole therapy surprisingly easy. Genuine feelings of hunger only occur infrequently and the physician is free to make decisions accordingly. "Starving" is not possible during therapy! However, it's another matter if food is not thoroughly chewed and insalivated, which is often the case. But this immediately corrects itself once proper eating habits have been learned.

2. Crisis

In the course of cleansing the colon and body, waste products may be abruptly resorbed into the bloodstream. This "retro-intoxication" of the organism by loosened debris is known as a crisis. This can be manifest by headaches, loss of appetite, aversion to eating or nausea, numbness, dizziness, moodiness and irritability, fatigue, feelings of weakness, vision problems, etc.

It usually comes on suddenly and lasts anywhere from minutes to hours, sometimes even days. Many patients, as well as their relatives, view these crises as a state of debilitation brought on by "undernourishment". Of course this is absolutely incorrect, because when the diet is resumed the patient always starts to feel well again. This happens as soon as the wave of toxins, which has inundated the body, has subsided and the poisonous material has been eliminated. The effect disappears with the cause.

However, reactions can occur in certain organs, in the form of "healing pains", for instance joints swell if pain in the joints was a pre-existing condition, or muscles ache in the case of persons with rheumatism, or pains in the gall bladder may occur if gall bladder disease was present. Pain can strike organs like the stomach, small or large intestine — especially the bends in the large intestine — or the ovaries if they were previously inflamed. But only organs that are not sound will have such a reaction. It can be an unpleasant surprise when organs thought to be healthy, suddenly respond painfully as they get better. The cause of such healing pains can be explained from the way chronic processes unfold: An acute and painful state of irritation (I) caused by damage to the organ, arises from an asymptomatic state of health (H). If this is not cured, it turns into a chronic state of paralysis (P). This is frequently asymptomatic because the nerve endings are paralysed by a kind of anesthesia.

H	→	**I**	→	**P**
Healthy condition	—	Irritation (Acute, painful)	—	Paralytic state (chronic) (often asymptomatic) (usually outwardly healthy)

P	→	**I**	→	**H**
Paralytic state	—	Irritation (painful)	—	Healthy condition

The way back follows the same route: The chronic stage returns to a state of irritation, becomes acute, (healing) pain occurs, until the final transition back into a state of health:

Healing powers activated by treatment monitor an organ's true state of health. Flare-ups of hidden foci of disease, which often occur just in time, and their elimination by therapy are particularly benefical.

Patients who bathe every day can graphically observe what's happening to their body during a crisis. Bath water that is otherwise relatively clean, is dirty on days when there is a crisis, and the bathtub has a grey ring around it*. This shows that considerable amounts of waste are being excreted by the skin. Other symptoms of a cleansing crisis are sweating, off-color, foul-smelling stools, bad breath and cloudy, acrid-smelling urine, and for women, temporary or increased vaginal discharge.

Besides intestinal debris, these various excretions contain toxins such as uric acid from the muscles, cholesterol from blood vessels, harmful bacteria and their poisons from lymph nodes, drugs and habit-forming toxins (nicotine!) stored in the body, and so on.

The best means of relief from a crisis are: MAT, drinking plenty of water, mineral water or herbal tea, skin brushing, alternating douches, bathing or washing, or taking a brisk walk in the fresh air. These help eliminate toxins rapidly and make the patient feel better.

3. Objective criteria for judging recovery

To correct a widespread misconception: changes in body weight are neither a basic nor a reliable criteria for good health. (During therapy thin people lose only a few pounds, while obese people usually experience a large weight loss).

On the other hand, Dr. *Mayr*'s diagnostics offer an objective indicator that monitors the body from top to bottom, pointing out the following unmistakable signs of improvement in overall health:

Facial muscles contract and tighten, signs of toxicity recede (see ill. 3), double chin and neck folds diminish, posture returns to normal (see ill. 2), with the neck assuming its normal shape and length, the distance between shoulder blades decreases, the lower thorax and hips become leaner, the abdomen softens and shrinks, a waist-

---

* Testing and verification of this phenomenon has been done by Dr. *Drumbl* from Graz.

line reappears, abnormal pelvic inclination corrects itself and the buttocks tucks in, spinal curvature decreases, and the body gets shapelier. The skin is a particularly good gauge of overall health. Its elasticity should eventually improve to the point where parts that hang — independent of weight loss or gain — noticeably pull up and become firm again. This sometimes happens several months after treatment has been completed. The worse the condition of the skin to begin with, the longer it will take to regenerate itself.

4. A few typical cases

Case history 4: Female physician, 28 years old, "duck" posture, loss of skin tone, became ill after childbirth from gallbladder disease. No improvement after being treated for 6 months by well-known physicians, constantly in pain, unable to work, has lost 33 lbs. (15 kg). In desperation, she underwent colon cleansing therapy under the direction of a student of Dr. *Mayr*'s. She was asymptomatic after only 5 weeks, could work again and had regained weight. The flaccid condition of her skin reverted to the puffy stage.

At the time, the author of this book was still working as a hospital-based physician and was very skeptical about any treatment not taught in medical school. However, as a result of this and other astonishing cures using Dr. *Mayr*'s method (he himself had been trained in it and even personally experienced its effectiveness), he decided to try it out on a few apparently desperate cases:

Case history 5: Postal official, 30, "Lazybones" posture, gall bladder removed 3 years ago, since then constant tenderness in the right upper abdomen; frequent, painful colic-like attacks. Patient spent 6 weeks in hospital and received almost daily injections of pain killers on the orders of the chief physician and others. No improvement despite various treatments, patient desperate. After being released, underwent *Mayr* therapy: No attacks after 10 days, regression of "liver hump", visible recovery. Completely asymptomatic after 6 weeks.

Case history 6: Owner of printing business, age 58, "bass drummer's" posture, skin in flaccid stage, in hospital for three weeks with angina-like symptoms, chest pains, fear of death, feeling of impending doom. No improvement despite intensive drug therapy, strict bed rest, etc. Since the attacks were brought on by elevation of the diaphram, the author tried manual abdominal treatment (MAT) in the region where opium-injections had been prescribed. After a few minutes all symptoms disappeared completely. Patient underwent *Mayr* therapy after being released from hospital: posture normalized, diaphram lowered (almost 10 cm!) and no more attacks. Completely symptom-free since then, without using any drugs; patient feels "born again".

Case history 7: Stenographer, female, age 35, "head-start" posture, 1st degree thinning of skin, recent stomach ulcer, 6-year-old duodenal ulcer. Since therapies and diets of all kinds had failed, sent to hospital to have ⅔ stomach removed (Billroth II op.). The author suggested trying *Mayr* therapy and patient requested leaving the hospital and having the operation postponed for 9 weeks. The physician in charge responded, "Go ahead, but you won't make it to the operating table". After 8 weeks in *Mayr* therapy, x-rays showed that the ulcers had already healed. Patient has been without relapse or symptoms for 8 years.

Case history 8: Professor, age 59, sower's posture, skin flaccid, serious damage to heart muscles, liver enlargement, edema, blood pressure 240, tinnitus, head congestion. Temporary improvement after 4-week hospital stay. 9 weeks after release, return of symptoms despite continued treatment. Instead of entering hospital again as ordered, patient underwent *Mayr* therapy, which lowered blood pressure to 155 and reversed cardiac dilation, liver enlargement and edema. Patient hasn't felt fitter or younger for years, takes *Mayr* therapy every year.

These and many other similar cases convinced the author that Dr. *Mayr*'s intestinal therapy was superior to traditional medical remedies. So he gave up the latter entirely to specialize in naturopathic inner body cleansing therapy. Since then, he has found that prescribing traditional drugs, including injections, has rarely been necessary.

Case history 9: Administrator, age 60, "bass drummer's" posture, skin flaccid, lips bluish, fatty degeneration of the heart muscle, enlarged liver, shortness of breath, nervousness. Under care of heart specialist for 5 years, mostly using injection therapy. Use of appetite suppressants and starvation diets were stopped each time because the patient became extremely nervous. Took *Mayr* therapy together with his wife and daughter. He didn't notice any hunger during the treatment and nervousness soon decreased (removal of nerve-stimulating intestinal toxins!). Heart symptoms and shortness of breath improve every day. Has lost 29 lbs. (12 kg) after 6 weeks of therapy, lips pink, all findings much better. Patient feels "at his peak".

Case history 10: Nun, age 28, "lazybones" posture, 2nd degree thinning of skin, sallow complexion, troubled by constipation since puberty, takes up to 10 (!) strong laxatives a day, but has bowel movement only once or twice a week, usually no relief with enemas, extremely painful abdominal cramps, eats almost nothing, vomits repeatedly every day. No basic improvement after 6 weeks' hospitalization. Since she wasn't from the area, she was given a leave to do *Mayr* therapy. After 3 weeks of strict treatment, daily bowel movements for the first time (still the wrong color and foul-smelling), could tolerate food, after 7 weeks abdomen soft, pain free, pink complexion, only 1st degree skin thinning, regular bowel movements. Gained 7 lbs. (3 kg) during therapy and another 9 lbs. (4 kg) afterwards.

Anemia present at the time greatly reduced and later cured during subsequent treatment. Patient completely fit again.

Case history 11: Housewife, age 38, "duck" posture, has had to use two canes for the past 6 month and walks with increasing difficulty. Back "very stiff", severe pains in small of back, radiating to both legs. Numerous injection treatments, several series of novocain infiltrates adminstered by specialists, treatments at health resorts, massages, etc. without any success. Patient desperate. In this case *Mayr* therapy was used in conjunction with special massages (gelotrypsy) for severe rheumatism of the soft tissues. (Massages are only effective if the deposits massaged out are evacuated with the stool and urine by revulsive "suction" produced by intestinal cleansing. Without this suction a large part of the toxins stirred up would remain in the body and gradually be redeposited.)

Patient is almost fully mobile after 8 weeks of treatment, agile and lively, symptoms return only when weather changes. X-rays show static normalization of the spinal column. Only the lumbar section of the spine was still out of line, which caused unsteadiness and weakness in the right leg. After chiropractic adjustment perfect mobility was restored and canes were never used again.

Case history 12: Publisher, 58, "sower's" posture, feels neither sick nor well. Loss of vitality, finds it hard to concentrate, "attacks of fatigue", suicidal feelings without specific cause. Regular bowel movements. Characteristic case of "autointoxication from intestines". No success from previous drug therapies. During treatment repeated crises with depression and even despair, alternating with days filled with optimism, joy and tremendous increase in work output. On crisis days looks wretched, even degenerate; complexion sallow. Elimination of foul-smelling, putrid, off-color masses of faeces. Still pale after 5 weeks in treatment but already extremely fit, 2 months after end of treatment healthy, upright posture, full of energy, free of depression.*

Case history 13: Salesperson, female, age 41, afflicted with boils for 2 years. They appeared one after the other — first on the neck, armpit and breast, then on the abdomen and particularly around the anus and external genitalia. Patient suicidal. 3 weeks in hospital, no cause could be determined; despite treatment there with diet, vitamin injections, penicillin, streptomycin, autochemotherapy and terramycin, new large boils still appeared. Finally cured after 9 weeks in *Mayr* therapy (without any other treatment).

Case history 14: Schoolgirl, 12, underdeveloped, increasingly anemic over a period of 2 years. Despite two hospital stays and subsequent treatment by a doctor from the mountain area where she lived, her red blood count fell to 2,560,000 and hemoglobin value to 50%. Examination using Dr. *Mayr*'s diagnostic system revealed severe damage to the ileum. (This meant that blood-building components from food could not be properly utilized by the body.) Constipation either went unnoticed or was "treated" with laxatives. After 4 weeks in *Mayr* therapy and 6 weeks on a transitional diet, 3,480,000

---

* In a scientific review of the above cases it states that the results could not be verified due to lack of stool and urinary records. However, since this was a paper intended for the general public, not doctors, results of analyses were purposely not given. In general, detailed analytical findings improve along with improvement in the patient's overall condition in *Mayr* therapy; besides, we are primarily concerned with the recovery of the sick person and not just an improvement in the "findings".

red blood corpuscles and Hb value 62%, after 3 more month 4,100,000 and Hb 72% and building toward eventual normalization.

Case history 15: Housewife, age 40, no children but had wanted a child for years. Left ovary removed because of cyst, right one full of adhesions. After gynocological examination, possibility of bearing children regarded hopeless. Inflammation of the small intestine and constipation were not noted, despite the fact that nourishment to sexual organs is transmitted through the small intestine. After 2 months in *Mayr* therapy with her husband, patient missed her period; 9 months later delivery of healthy girl.*

Our dear friends

In this world, there are both reasonable and unreasonable people. Unfortunately the latter are probably more numerous. Those who don't know this yet, quickly learn it the moment they tell their acquaintances they have started inner body cleansing.

The *know-it-all,* unencumbered by knowledge of the facts, feels immediately obliged to raise a warning cry. Since he has eaten ever since he was born and since he has also been hungry, he considers himself an expert on "starvation diets"**. He can therefore offer the best advice, better at least than any doctor.

The overly-cautious react negatively: "You won't be able to make it!" "You'll lose too much weight, get attacks of nerves...!" and so on.

Malicious people are pessimistic: "Eating like that will give you TB or cancer!" "You're digging your own grave — you'll get ulcers from lack of vitamins ..."

The *"well-meaning neighbor",* who forces a "special meal" on the zealous faster, takes the opposite tack: "This can't do any harm", she

---

* Such cases are not rare. Sexually underdeveloped women or women whose sexual organs have been damaged are able to conceive more easily after therapy because their genitals are healthy. The effect of this treatment can be documented by *Kuhne* friction sitz-baths.

** The term "starvation diet" to describe *Mayr* therapy is wrong on many counts, especially since, if done correctly, starving is never experienced at all.

whispers in the sweetest voice and is tickled to death her temptation succeeds. It wouldn't be entirely fair to say she is pleased by someone else's misfortune, it's just that her maternal instinct to feed and a senseless sort of "empathy" overwhelm her.

But the worst are people who are overweight themselves. Overcome by jealousy at the sight of someone getting slimmer, they make thinly-veiled comments about "this dangerous treatment".

Students of history know that the reaction of contemporaries to innovative ideas, especially if they affect comfortable habits, is usually strenuous opposition. So it's no surprise that the new intestinal cleansing treatment should be controversial: it breaks the hold that "eating" and the pursuit of pleasure have over us and destroys our illusion that true recovery can be achieved effortlessly.

Although statistics from life insurance companies have long shown the opposite, the idea that "a rounded appearance" is the same as a "healthy appearance" is still generally believed. So people become concerned, even annoyed, when the person doing *Mayr* therapy loses his layer of fat, double chin and pot belly, thus giving the lie to the conventional "ideal of healthiness" by his "poor appearance".

But since neither unreasonable nor tactless people are going to disappear tomorrow, it would be wise to discuss the program only with those whose support can be relied on.

Happily there are also reasonable people. They known that their relatives or friends are under a doctor's orders; as laymen they won't interfere except to help you stick with the requirements of the treatment.

Very reasonable people even taken the treatment with you. Success doubles when an entire family decides to do *Mayr* therapy together. The experience solidifies a group; housekeeping is simplified and noticably easier financially. The latter applies to the future too, because people who have regained their health through this program usually end up eating less.

What such a streamlined eating plan would mean to a whole population has yet to be determined. If people gave up their bad eating habits, the resulting improvement in health could bring about an overall rise in efficiency and production at work. Billions of dollars now spent on junk foods could be saved; the enormous amount spent on drugs and therapeutic diets, hospital care and other social programs would be reduced and countless millions of man hours, now lost in the workplace due to diet-related illness, could be used in the production of goods. Dr. *Mayr* goes into detail about this in his works and foresees unsuspected new horizons.

Mayr therapy is most beneficial when married couples cleanse themselves internally before producing any offspring. Reproductive organs are able to regenerate and damaging substances can be expelled before they are passed on to the next generation. The mother's body as a future home is thoroughly clean before being inhabited by a new being, and the mother's blood, for 9 months the only source of life for the baby, is purified. the result is better prenatal development and better milk production by the mother.

Inner body cleansing ought to become mandatory for aware young women.

Vitamins and drugs

During the lean years of the last war, millions of people's ailments disappeared, even long-standing ones; there was a dramatic decline in the number of patients under treatment. According to health department statistics, this "healthy period" came to an end soon after normal conditions returned, and the old complaints caused by a rich, fatty diet, high in sugar, again cropped up in large numbers: angina pectoris, high blood pressure and stroke, arterial sclerosis, diseases of the stomach and gall bladder, obesity, gout, diabetes, gynecological and hormonal problems became more and more frequent and have now turned into the scourge of civilized man.

Natural sources of vitamins are again abundant. But as long as overeating and gourmet meals are the order of the day, all the vitamin-rich foods in the world will not be able to check the downward spiral of people's health. On the contrary. Swamping the body with vitamins is an exercise in futility. The modern addiction to vitamins (bowls of salad and mountains of fruit every day) encouraged by advertising and health food advocates produces — and this is very little known — manifold damage to health. Using Dr. *Mayr*'s diagnostics, this can be seen in the intestines (irritation, gas), the liver (enlargement), blood vessels (dilation and capillary paralysis) and other organs. Large amounts of raw foods decompose in the intestines, particularly, of course, in the intestines of people who suffer from diseases of the digestive tract. People who eat raw foods exclusively even end up with the same bluish-red nose and ears as alcoholics. Eating too many raw foods causes them to ferment in the intestines like grapes in a mash tub, forming alcohol-fusel toxins that go about their daily work unnoticed. The widespread notion that one cannot possibly get too many vitamins is as ill-concieved as the opinion that one cannot expose oneself to too much sun. Aside from the fact that *the right number of vitamins is available naturally,* the health of the intestines is the crux of the whole vitamin issue.

Healthy people need only a small number of vitamins. There is no deficiency during Mayr therapy, since, in our experience, the absorbability of the intestines improves so much that the amount found in the foods eaten is sufficient. In fact,

During therapy, taking extra vitamins in the form of fruit juices, pills, etc. is considered bad practice and is strictly prohibited!

The intestines have to rest at this time and learn how to ration themselves for later. Intestinal flora, which produce numerous vitamins like B1, B2, biotin, niacinamide, folic acid and B12, as well as vitamin K and others, also recover as therapy progresses. The following cases attest to this:

Case history 16: Female, 45, had only eaten raw foods for years, came for treatment complaining of constantly bleeding gums. Diagnosis: Severe lack of vitamin C, extremely slack intestines (!). Patient took only milk, rolls and tea, in addition to the juice of a half a lemon daily, a fraction of the amount of vitamin C taken previosly in her daily diet. After 3 weeks' respite, no more spontaneous bleeding of gums, after 4 weeks not even when brushing teeth. Completely cured after 6 weeks of treatment.

Cases like this can help us to view the question of vitamins in a completely different light.

The well-known health activist *Werner Zimmermann,* who had been a great advocate of eating uncooked foods, comments on the above section:

"We had similar experiences in 1960 when we — my wife, a few friends and I — entered Mayr therapy. We met three young women who for 10 years had lived their lives in strict accordance with the teachings of *Bircher, Kollath* and *Waerland.* They were trying to get over some particularly stubborn ailments. Two of them suffered from chronic excema, the third from bleeding gums. After only a few days in Mayr therapy they all showed improvement. Nervous children stopped having gas, they slept better and woke happier. What I saw obliges me to come out publically in favor of this new approach. We have to constantly re-examine what we believe."

Addiction to pills

The right medicine, correctly used, effectively supports a person's recovery, assuming that he also gives up his bad habits.

However, many people expect to be cured solely by drugs, without ever doing anything themselves. They are usually disappointed in the long run. True, symptoms are either suppressed or deadened as long as medication is being taken, but the disease is still present and may even get worse. This is the way lots of people become chemically dependent; they think they can't live any more without some pill or other. Once their bodies adjust to a certain dosage, they have to increase their intake. But the constant consumption of sundry pills turns the advantage of prescription drugs into the curse of drug addiction. Chronic poisoning that produces organic damage (digestive and blood diseases, allergies, etc.) or functional disturbances of the nervous system are common consequences. For instance, in 1954 in Austria alone, people took:

80 million painkillers, 30 million aspirin, 40 million sleeping pills, 50 million laxative tablets, and so on. In West Germany today, 35,000 different prescription drugs are in common use. In England 1.75 billion tranquilizers are used annually[*].

These figures should be enough to illustrate the shocking dimensions of a method of treating illness that is totally out of proportion, that indeed gives into the demands of the average person not to forego any convenience, even temporarily, and *runs completely counter to the real needs of a sick organism.*

---

[*] Österr. Ärzteztg. 18/IX. 1958. These figures have increased rapidly every year until now (1970). And even today (1986) they continue to increase steadily.

Health insurance companies are trying to combat this abuse of drugs, along with its very serious public health and economic consequences, by making it more difficult to obtain certain prescription drugs. But they are barking up the wrong tree.

Only early education about good eating habits and healthy lifestyles, and the promotion of natural healing, which eliminates the necessity of prescribing and using drugs for often minor reasons, can end this abuse and improve public health. This would make it impossible for health insurance companies to run up million dollar deficits for the cost of medication for flu epidemics. Most cases of flu can be cured without medication anyway, by using herbs, hydrotherapy and sweatbaths. On the other hand, the consumption of medication is enormous when tonics and pills alone are used to treat cold symptoms and then later other medications have to be taken to undo the damage of the first medicine (for instance, stomach-intestinal upsets, gastritis, abnormal bacterial flora, liver damage, allergies). Dr. *Mayr*'s health precepts follow a completely different line of thinking in this matter*.

Conclusion of therapy and repetition

Often the hardest part of therapy is letting it gradually come to a successful end. It's particularly important at this time not to relax and get careless, but to remain conscientious about keeping all the rules and to chew and insalivate even more thoroughly than before. Even the smallest deviations in diet and eating are noticable now. The mucous membranes, which have just been rejuvenated, are still tender and respond with an intense feeling of soreness to unwholesome foods, such as those containing "scouring" cellulose. Particularly stubborn cases are sometimes just coming into the crisis stage at this point. Such patients — instead of becoming resigned and discouraged — must understand the reason for this and work very

---

* One would assume that health insurance companies would support those who use natural healing methods like *Mayr* therapy. For reasons of economics alone, it would be in the interest of insurance companies if a significant number of patients being treated were basically healthier and didn't have to take numerous and expensive drugs. Unfortunately these connections are often completely missed.

conscientiously to get even better results. During this transitional period the doctor will try to determine the needs of each individual patient and make up a diet the patient can follow in the future. The goal is to end up with a nutritional plan that is best for each patient.

Food preparation is also very important at this point. The foods and their preparation described in the book *Modified Diet for Effective Elimination* have been specifically designed for the smoothest possible transition from a stricter diet and are especially good for people with sensitive stomachs and intestines. Rather than devouring large amounts of food, it's important to remember that savoring each bite will be pleasurable. Quality should replace quantity. Now more than ever the instinct, the desire for specific, simple, natural foods will emerge and it should be heeded. Meals that were once favorites, such as heavily marbled beef, bacon, baked goods and candy, desserts, and sophisticated gourmet dishes may be turned down. Chocolate, alcohol, liquor, and coffee lose their appeal as one's body becomes healthier. The conclusion of therapy determines its success and lays the groundwork for better eating habits in the future.

Repeating therapy

Though Mayr therapy has proven very successful in curing some of the most difficult cases, its main purpose should lie in repeating it for the sake of preventing illness and maintaining good health. Prevention is always better than a cure! People should regularly — once a year in most cases — clean and invigorate their internal organs with intestinal therapy, just as they routinely wash and clean the outside of their bodies.

Dangers of self-treatment

It would not occur to most people to operate on their own ulcer, to set their own bones or to cure their heart disease by reading a medical textbook. Yet many lay people undertake drastic diet and nutritional therapies by themselves because they think they are dealing with something simple and harmless. However, they overlook the fact that this type of treatment has long been a medical specialty — and for good reason because, even more than other types of therapy, it influences the organism fundamentally and goes directly to the heart of most problems. Thus it requires special experience and knowledge, since even something beneficial, if incorrectly applied, can also do just as much harm.

There are already too many people who have gotten innocently caught in dangerous undertakings by reading things like "The Waerland diet saved us!"; after an initial improvement, they often found themselves in catastrophic circumstances.

The dangers of another incorrectly administered diet therapy, which three general *physicians* did on their own, was recently reported in a medical journal, along with its disasterous consequences.

The same goes of course for Mayr therapy.

For this reason, we repeat the following case of someone who undertook his own Mayr treatment and did it incorrectly:

Male, 42, decided, on the basis of a story told him by a friend, to undergo inner body cleansing on his own. After 24 days of feeling very good, he became somewhat weak and tired (crisis!). He took this as a sign that therapy was over, went immediately to a restaurant and ate his favorite dish, cucumber salad (!), That night, painful cramps, internal bleeding, admitted to hospital. ⅔ of stomach removed.

In this and unfortunately many other cases of self-treatment, permanent damage was done instead of a permanent improvement. This would not have happened if therapy had been properly directed. Therefore *Mayr therapy must only be done under the direction of a trained physician.* This may necessitate a stay at a health resort. However, those who, for whatever reason, cannot take a cure or cannot do it correctly, should pay particular attention to the suggestions in the following section.

Part III

Better nutrition and a healthier way of life

Proper nutrition

All the books and papers that have been written on the subject of nutrition in the past decade could fill a library all by themselves. Not a day goes by that the results of new research and testing are not published*.

Yet opinions on the subject are scattered all over the map. If one were to avoid all the foods that at one time or another were thought to be dangerous to our health, one would have to go hungry in front of a full plate.

This is also true for the maze of nutritional systems, diet fads and therapies. Objectively speaking, i.e. measured according to *Mayr*'s signs of good health (compare ill. 2 and 3), they are seldom successful in the long run, and probably never could be because they cannot produce the prerequisite for proper nutrition, namely a healthier (i.e. cleaned and completely efficient) digestive system, and most people don't have one to start with. *Nutrition*, states Dr. *Mayr*, cannot be equated with *food*. According to the formula:

$$N\text{utrition} = F\text{ood} \times D\text{igestion}$$

nutrition is the product of the Food Factor times the Digestion Factor. But as long as the Digestion Factor is flawed, the body can never be completely nourished. Therefore the digestive system *has to be made sound before better nourishment of the organism can take place.* Along with this recuperation, the natural mechanisms governing proper nourishment have to be released from their state of atrophy or pathological deformation.

---

* The periodical "Nutrition Abstracts and Reviews" reports on 16,000 works published annually on nutrition-related issues.

Just as animals living in the wild without any knowledge of nutritional systems are able to feed themselves so well that their lifespans go well beyond their period of growth, man also possesses faculties which help him *select the right foods and regulate their intake:*

1. Food selectors

a) **Sight** draws us to that which is naturally colorful, healthy, ripe and fresh, and steers us away from what is ugly, unripe, shrivelled, aged and spoiled. Thus we prefer apples which are rosy-red and golden yellow, strawberries that are dark red and huckleberries that are blue-black, over their unripe, inconspicuous neighbors. The benefit of evaluating food with our sense of sight has been damaged irreparably because so many fresh foods are now chemically dyed and "cosmetically" treated (chemically dyed oranges, lemons; vegetables kept artificially fresh-looking, etc.). Nevertheless, we should remember that fresh, ripe, unprocessed foods are always best for us. Thus lettuce picked from the garden and served immediately is healthier than lettuce that finds its way to the table via wholesalers and retailers.

b) **Smell** draws us to food that smells good, that makes our mouths water, and warns us against unpleasant-smelling things that are dangerous and decomposing. If our sense of smell were as powerful today as it formerly was, it would automatically "turn on" so much while food was being prepared that most cooking (particularly what is known as home cooking!) would have to improve. After Mayr therapy one's sense of smell is more acute and should be paid close attention to. Anyone with a keener sense of smell will reject dishes that don't smell right: slightly spoiled or chemically prepared foods, e.g. chemically-fertilized cabbage, coarse cauliflower, some kinds of meat, etc.

c) **Touch** by the hands, the lips, teeth and tongue tells us more about the consistency of foods; our sense of touch warns us if something is either too hot or too cold. Numerous cases of stomach-intestinal illness are due to the fact that our sense of temperature has been dulled (gastritis, enteritis from drinking ice-cold drinks).

d) **Taste** indicates the properties of sweet, sour, bitter, salty and their mixtures, subjects foods to a final test, and advises us whether to eat something or reject it. Neither chain smokers nor alcoholics can count themselves among those whose sense of taste is reliable, nor can gourmands who love eating unwholesome foods, roasts and gravies dripping with fat, sugary foods, jams and jellies, etc.; likewise no healthy person would ever think of judging life only by the motto "we live to eat", as is so common today.

The weaker our senses are, the less instinctive and more aberrant will be our food choices, the more confused our attitude toward many aspects of life in general. Finally, many people get sick — both physically and mentally — because only what is bad and unhealthy tastes good to them.

But healthy senses don't need to be either compelled or forbidden.

The more discriminating the senses are made by regular intestinal therapy, the easier it is for someone to tell what he ought and what he ought not to eat.

Whatever applies to the senses also applies to:

2. The protective reflexes of the digestive system as regulators of food intake

a) **The satiation reflex** tells the body when it has had enough food. Neither too much nor too little, but just the right amount is beneficial to good health. Only a correctly functioning satiation reflex can best control human nutrition. Unfortunately, this is the reflex that is so dulled or so irritated in the average person that they almost never eat the right amount. (See p. 72 "How much should we eat?").

b) **The swallowing reflex** prevents us from swallowing bites that have not been sufficiently broken down in the oral cavity. These it projects forward again to be chewed and insalivated more thoroughly. After satiation, it also prevent any more swallowing. This is demonstrated when healthy infants spit out their food.

c) **The gag reflex** serves as a protection for the stomach and intestines by regurgitating food that has been swallowed but not chewed, is too big or is otherwise dangerous. A gag reflex that has been dulled only reacts to blatantly harmful situations, such as fish bones, sharp bone fragments, excessively spicey or hot dishes, acids, lyes, etc. taken by mistake, or if food starts to go down "the wrong tube".

If our swallowing and gag reflexes had not become so dulled, our *meal*times, in which bites are supposed to be thoroughly *ground* by the teeth, would never have turned into the quick affairs they often are now.

d) The vomiting reflex also protects the body by throwing harmful food back into the mouth. Its development from the nursing infant who can still vomit, through older children who only just feel awful, to the adult celebrant, who can get through a sumptuous (and harmful) banquet without a hitch, demonstrates just how this protective reflex becomes dulled. This is by no means a positive development, for if isolated damage cannot be immediately dealt with, we will later be presented with a whopping final bill that cannot be paid.

Contrary to what is generally thought, a healthy stomach is not necessarily one that does not react to bad eating habits. People with so-called "cast iron stomachs" are precisely the ones who often develop stomach troubles.

Both the senses and the protective reflexes of the digestive system *can only function correctly in an organism cleaned by repeated intestinal therapy. This results in an improved nutritional condition that has a positive effect on health and outlook on life.*

Eating right

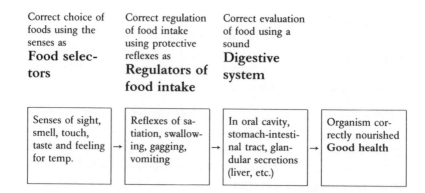

Correct choice of foods using the senses as **Food selectors**	Correct regulation of food intake using protective reflexes as **Regulators of food intake**	Correct evaluation of food using a sound **Digestive system**	
Senses of sight, smell, touch, taste and feeling for temp. →	Reflexes of satiation, swallowing, gagging, vomiting →	In oral cavity, stomach-intestinal tract, glandular secretions (liver, etc.) →	Organism correctly nourished **Good health**

How should we eat?

Horace Fletcher was an American salesman, who by the age of 40 was unable to work and practically senile. His application for life insurance had been turned down. Various medical treatments brought no improvement. Then, on the advice of a friend who enjoyed particularly good health, he began to chew and insalivate all his food so thoroughly that it was liquified by the time it reached his stomach. To achieve this he chewed approximately 2,500 times per meal*.

Gradually his esophagous refused to let anything pass that had not been well chewed and insalivated (his swallowing and gagging reflex improved) and he felt satisfied with less food (his satiation reflex improved). This satisfaction also lasted longer. His desire for high-protein foods, spicy dishes, for sweets, alcohol, coffee and tea decreased and he preferred a variety of simple, natural foods (his selectors improved). Concerned friends** were alarmed by *Fletcher's* loss of weight and told him he didn't look good. But *Fletcher* stuck with it. After 5 months of disciplined chewing, all his complaints had disappeared and his sense of well-being was at an all-time high. He was setting records for strength and endurance when he was 50, even 60 years old, and this on 1600 calories a day, instead of the officially recommended 3400! Tests by several scientists and nutrition specialists showed that his metabolism was well-balanced and that he had outstanding muscle tone and endurance***.

Since results like *Fletcher's* cannot be expected in every case, we cannot objectively recommend this regimen. However, the fact remains that *simply chewing and insalivating food more thoroughly relieves the digestive system and thus brings about a fundamental improvement in overall health.*

Moreover, eating correctly goes hand in hand with inner peace and a homey atmosphere. A wife should never talk about her vexations, worries and needs until after the meal and a husband should

---

* *Fletcher, Horace:* "How I Became Young at 60".
** See section entitled "Our dear friends" on p. 59.
*** Examined by Prof. *Foster* and Prof. *Gowland-Hopkins* of Cambridge Univ., Prof. *Pickering-Bowditsch* and Prof. *Chittenden* of Yale Univ., Prof. *Fisher,* and others, according to *Fletcher.*

likewise postpone any adverse criticism of the meal until later. Constant talk distracts people from the task of eating and causes them to bolt their food down. Eating while working, reading, watching TV or as a means of suppressing anger is harmful!

Eight rules for eating right

1. *Take enough time.*
   At least 1/2 hour!
2. *Serve foods attractively.*
3. *Eat slowly, in comfort and liesure.*
4. *Take small bites.*
5. *Chew carefully and insalivate every bite.*
   Food well chewed is food half digested.
6. *Savor every bite.*
7. *Concentrate on eating.*
   Free yourself from distractions and disturbances (Newspaper, conversation, television = poison!)
8. *Make sure the bite on false teeth is aligned.*
   Good dentures are better than your own bad teeth!

How much should we eat?

> Cows know when it is time to go home
> And willingly leave their grassy trough
> But unwise men
> Never know when
> Their stomachs are full enough.
>
> The Edda

The following words were written on Egyptian papyrus 5700 years ago:

"Most people eat too much. They thrive on a quarter of what they eat and the physicians thrive from the other three quarters."

And the Roman writer and naturalist *Pliny* wrote:

"Most people work to fill their bellies, which then cause them untold suffering."

Nothing has changed since then.

Everyone requires a different amount of food. How much is determined by various individual factors like digestion (utilization of foods), physical and mental work, age, sex, etc. But the amount that is right for each person can only be indicated by a properly functioning satiation reflex. But this reflex is usually jaded, so the average eater can no longer rely on his feeling of when to stop, but usually keeps on eating until he is full. This no longer has anything to do with a sound satiation reflex.

Moderation should be the basis for evaluating how much we eat. If people chewed their food well, they would soon be able to recognize what the right amount of food is for them. *Mayr* therapy is an excellent way to awaken this satiation reflex. Surprisingly people usually end up eating very little, and for some, half of what they ate before is sufficient. *Horace Fletcher* was even able to get along on only a third.

But there are also people who don't eat enough. By rehabilitating their digestive organs, they too can learn to sense the amount of food needed by their bodies.

Problems about how much to eat first surface when

a child's natural appetite is upset.

We can observe this phenomenon in its two extremes — the corpulent child who is always ravenous, and the sickly child with no appetite. A genetic predisposition, illness or a chaotic environment may be to blame, but *mostly it's due to blatent errors in feeding* infants, toddlers and schoolchildren.

Aside from a specific illness, such as adenoids, chronic inflammation of the tonsils, catarrh, worms, sluggish bowels accompanied by constipation, etc., chronic lack of appetite is primarily present in children who were always made to eat and had the painful experience of *having* to eat instead of *wanting* to eat. The more eating was forced upon them, the more resistant they became.

Children shouldn't be asked again and again if they want more to eat. The less we concern ourselves with how much a child eats, the more naturally and freely what he eats will conform to what his body needs. Children who eat at the family table should be given small portions; they can always ask for more.

On the other hand, sweets, candy, or snacks given during or between meals will exaccerbate any existing digestive disturbance, ruin a normal appetite and damage the stomach, intestinal flora, teeth and bones (posture!). Too many sweets also produce a tendency toward illness, laziness, lack of concentration, nervousness, bad moods, and small but numerous deficiencies in physical and mental development.

Chronic lack of appetite in children can also be caused by unwillingness to chew. This is promoted by eating puréed foods, which don't require chewing and insalivating. Irregular mealtimes, lack of fresh air, tiredness after school, family quarrels, incorrect handling of children (lack of parental understanding) and withholding love will cause a child to lose his appetite and retard development.

Mayr therapy, adapted to each individual, but with an absolute "no sweets" rule, has proven very effective against such disturbances, assuming that the other causes mentioned have been ruled out or taken care of. Findings have shown how necessary intestinal cleansing is even for children and how rapidly their bodies respond to it. With reasonable supervision, children quite willingly keep the rules of the treatment, even those who were addicted to junk food. The fact that children's instincts are not as dulled contributes to this success.

When and how often should we eat?

So then until philosophy
Holds together land and sea,
Life continues well enough
Through hunger and through love.
Schiller

Hunger, that powerful, primordial urge, makes the need for food known to the body. Those who can distinguish real hunger from its false brother — a pathological need to eat and an appetite for sweets — live by the Chinese wiseman *Laotse*'s dictum:

"Eat when you are hungry and drink when you are thirsty!
But remember, anything more will only do you harm!"

For them the thought of simple foods, like good bread, a glass of milk or a ripe, juicy apple makes their mouths water. They don't think about their favorite dish or delicacies, but are completely content with simple, unprocessed foods. *Since genuine hunger expresses a natural desire to eat, it is never accompanied by severe discomfort.*

On the other hand, ravenousness, abdominal pressure, a painful empty feeling in the stomach and intestines, hunger pains, nausea, dizziness and sudden weakness are all signs of illness. These are symptoms of an unhealthy, false hunger and are not caused by lack of food, but by autointoxication of the intestinal system. If food is not eaten at the usual time, an unhealthy intestinal system is forced to work on intestinal contaminants; this releases toxic substances into the blood stream and leads to the above symptoms. Once the person eats again, only the new food is processed, while the intestinal contaminants remain in place. This causes autointoxication and its symptoms to retreat. So these people eat all the time in order to satisfy their apparent hunger, which is in truth a symptom of illness. They think they are starving to death if they haven't eaten anything for a few hours. But this is not true.

As their health improves during intestinal cleansing therapy, they are no longer tortured by false hunger, get to know what real hunger feels like and learn when and how often they should actually eat to nourish themselves.

The better their digestive organs get, the better they can judge what foods are good to eat, and the less they need to eat. In the end, two main meals are enough; eating between meals is not only superfluous, but even adverse.

As to the question of

the evening meal

Dr. *Mayr* says the following: "Eating a substantial meal before going to bed is like a train conductor who stokes up his engine and then puts it in the round house."

As everyone knows, sleeping at night has the function of restoring energy to the body. The activity of all the organs slows down, breathing and digestive processes continue at a slower pace. Thus dinner sits undigested in the warm, damp digestive tract for hours, fermenting or becoming spoiled by bacterial action, inviting narcotic-like toxins to enter the circulatory system. Large amounts of food initially produce a state of excitement (tossing and turning, waking up repeatedly, bad dreams), then later toward morning a state of sluggishness (leaden sleep, relaxation of soft palate so that one snores, relaxation of the jaw muscles so that the mouth gapes open and saliva covers the pillow). Instead of waking bright and fresh in the morning, such people wake up slowly, dazed and exhausted, as though they were hung over from a night of drinking. The mirror reveals a pale, wretched-looking face, with eyes glued shut, a dry, sticky taste in the mouth, and disheveled hair.

A few nights without dinner produces the opposite effect! Sleep is peaceful and deep, waking is joyful and refreshing.

Thus Dr. *Mayr* generally advises against eating an evening meal. Instead he recommends herbal tea with lemon or honey. This may be accompanied by a piece of stale white bread (because it's easily digested), with or without a spread (a little butter, cottage cheese, white cheese or the like), or a soft boiled egg.

Foods that ferment easily and are hard to digest, like fruit (an apple is "gold in the morning, silver at noon, and lead at night!"), vegetables, legumes and fresh yeast products are especially bad when eaten in large quantities late in the evening.

Only those who are genuinely hungry at night because they are processing their food efficiently should eat — though not too late and only a little of something that is easy to digest. And this should be well chewed. A walk afterwards is highly recommended for stimulating the digestive processes and for improving the quality of sleep.

What should we eat?

What's good for the goose
Is bad for the gander.

Folk saying

This bit of folk wisdom can refer to the fact that there is no universal type of nutrition. "The man that works like a thresher should eat like a thresher", says Dr. *Mayr*. "But those who don't work like threshers" — and very few work that hard now — "can't eat like threshers." This refers to both the quality and the quantity of food. Someone who works hard, especially out of doors, needs more and different kinds of food, foods more difficult to digest, than someone who works indoors in an office.

People who have gone through inner body cleansing therapy have no desire to return to their old eating habits. They want better nutrition in the future. To achieve this we should enjoy each bite of food we take. Rather than thinking of quantity by gorging ourselves, by eating quickly or nervously, we should be thinking of quality by savoring small portions, using, eating habits recently gained through therapy, training and refinement of our senses. This way everyone can find out for himself what foods he needs, what his digestive system can handle and thus what is right for him. This newly awakened eating instinct responds to *simple, healthy, unprocessed, uncombined foods,* not old favorite dishes and sweets. This genuine need should be heeded, dismissing any and all theories about food: don't keep eating a bland diet, dry rolls or white bread just because they worked during therapy; stop hankering after certain vitamin-rich foods because vitamins are supposed to be "good for you"; and forget about counting calories or consulting other lists! Individual nutritional needs and the benefits of these foods will be reliable indicators of what the organism requires. Aside from individual deviations, and depending of course on individual digestive systems, *a varied diet not based on one type of food, should generally be used as a permanent diet:* milk and milk products, including cottage cheese and cream cheese; crusty old black bread; root or leaf vegetables, like carrots, parsley, black salsify, lettuce, celery, salads, spinach and other kinds of unprocessed vegetables, prepared in the "English style" if possible; potatoes; fruits like apples or berries, plain or with milk, in the morning or before lunch; grain products like oatmeal, rice, hominy grits, millet, perhaps with soy sauce; also eggs, fish, lean meat (veal, chicken, beef). This diet can then be varied or expanded according to personal needs. People who don't want to eat meat should stay away from it, those who do, should eat it without hesitation. Their bodies probably need it.

The best fruits are berries (huckleberries, strawberries, raspberries), followed by apples and bananas (if not sprayed!); last and least beneficial are the stone fruits (cherries, plums, apricots, etc.), which decompose readily. Generally speaking, however, raw foods should only be eaten in moderation. If only a little bit more is eaten than the intestines can manage (for instance of cherries, pears, lettuce, cabbage etc.), rampant fermentation will occur in the intestines. This means the formation of fusel, damage to the liver and vascular system and autointoxication, accompanied by burping, rumbling stomach, colic, abdominal distention and toxic flatulence.

Raw juices are not recommended because they also ferment easily. They are usually drunk too quickly anyway, so they don't get mixed well with saliva. Dr. *Mayr* says, if drinking juice were meant to be nature's way of consuming fruit, we would have had beaters in our mouths instead of teeth.

Generally speaking, local fruit is preferred over produce from abroad that is picked green and grown in unknown soils.

The more active the ingredients in a food product, the more quickly a large quantity can destroy the value of good quality. Therefore, always use moderation, especially when eating raw foods!

"Home cooking" can also be harmful because of its high caloric content and because ingredients are usually cooked to death. It relies on daily consumption of meat; lavish use of lard or fat; roasts, rouxs, grilled meats; and frying everything, even vegetables; it also includes lots of pasta, noodles and dumplings, in addition to pastries and other sweet desserts.

To be avoided:

1. Using too much fat in roasting, rouxs, frying (vegetables should also be steamed "English style"), as well as anything that contains a lot of fat (use butter and oil sparingly, and don't use pork fat at all! —

2. Anything very sweet (sweets are harmful, produce fermentation toxins, tooth decay, destroy calcium, and rob the body of vitamin B. Keep away from sugar, especially children! Honey is healthier, but it too should be used in moderation.) —

3. Anything that "fights back", is hard to process, produces gas or irritates the colon (stool too soft, soiled anus etc.), for instance, tough vegetables, legumes, fresh or very dense breads, large amounts of fruit or fruit juices —

4. Fresh baked goods —

5. Eating different foods at the same time or several courses one after another —

6. Stale or leftover foods (e.g. a housewife eating the proverbial leftovers for lunch).

It is also wrong to:

eat when not genuinely hungry —
eat in a hurry —
eat when physically or mentally tired (rest up first).

In contrast, **new eating habits** are maintained following intestinal therapy by:
eating quietly and in leisure —
chewing and insalivating thoroughly —
savoring every single bite (only things that taste better after being chewed 50 times are good for you) —
refining one's sense of pleasure —
taking moderate portions (especially of live foods) —
preparing foods simply and naturally.

General rules for good health:

The three basic principles of respite, cleansing and training are extremely important for improving digestion and serve as overall rules for a healthier life.

1. Respite

Sleep at night, the resting and recuperative phase most important to humans, serves to renew the body's energy. The deep sleep before midnight is the most beneficial, Thus:

Go to bed early and at the same time every night!

Again, tiredness is a signal that it is time to stop our activities. If this signal is not heeded, we enter the stage of fatigue. Granted, this can be driven off by will power or with stimulants like coffee, alcohol, chain smoking or drugs; but if this is repeated often enough it leads into a labyrinth of chronic fatigue, out of which it is not easy to find one's way. Many urbanites are caught in this trap, without the strength to liberate themselves even for a few hours from the nerve-wracking daily grind. Ambition, craving for recognition, extreme aquisitiveness, addiction to eating and drinking, and other obsessive and confused lifestyles that turn night into day (watching TV constantly, too!) take away inner peace, reason and repose. The effects on the autonomic nervous system are many and varied. They range all the way from slight disturbances (dystonia), which can produce symptoms in all the organs, to psychosomatic complaints, like depression, anxiety, heart, sleep and sexual dysfunction, to death itself in the prime of life. The sense of life becomes nonsense. *Maladjustment to life has now unquestionably become the primary source of illness.*

How few know the answer to the wiseman's question:

*"You are always rushing around, my friend. Where are you going in such a hurry?"**

How few bother with the deeper meaning they could give their lives! They have lost any re-ligio, or re-attachment to a higher source of life or is it only a figment of their imaginations. Those who lack this deeper conviction also lack any order in their lives, lack the impetus for creative work, joy, feelings of happiness, harmony and also — health. In this case only an inner reorientation — discovering the higher meaning in one's own existence — can bring about the change necessary for healing. Hence, the saying goes: "Do not ask what is the meaning of your life, but rather how you can give meaning to your life"**. Only those who are willing to look for it will find it!

The intricate interplay between spiritual outlook and psycho-organic function is just now being understood at a time when inner rootlessness, haste and unrest are so prevelant that anyone genuinely wanting to recuperate has to deal with it: Only those who look into themselves can create inner order. Mental chaos and stress lead to illness and suffering:

Hurt feelings lead to chest pains,
Worry and care to sleeplessness and nervous breakdown,
Unsolved problems to stomach and intestinal ulcers,
Irritation to gall bladder attacks,
Constant stress to heart attack,
Outbreaks of anger to stroke.

Thus great importance is attached to mental relaxation and order. Balance in one's daily activities is beneficial in many respects: mod-

* *Bo Yin Ra* in *The Path to God.*
** *Bo Yin Ra, The Meaning of Existence*

erate involvement in sports, hiking through the woods and mead-
ows, gardening, bowling, fishing and other hobbies which afford ac-
cess to the outdoors and a positive change of pace; reading good
books, listening to music, doing crafts, having meaningful conversa-
tions — aside from their intrinsic merits — also let one forget the
daily routine, gain perspective and help an individual to bear life's
burdens better, not taking them quite so seriously. People relax and
recuperate, the wear and tear of daily life stops and they regain their
resiliency.

2. Cleansing

Anything that makes our cleaned and decontaminated organs
work better improves metabolism. Some of these things are:

a) Daily bathing

Mathias Zdarsky, an Austrian pioneer of good health habits, made
the following remark: "People who think of themselves as very clean,
state with pride that they wash from the waist up every day. The
lower half is on lease to the perfume factory."

During cleansing therapy, but otherwise too, taking showers alternating with hot and cold water or washing all over with a cold or
lukewarm washcloth is recommended. By doing this, one part of the
body after another is well rubbed down. The washcloth should be
repeatedly squeezed out and dipped in fresh water. After washing in
the evening, it's best to leave the skin slightly damp and immediately
put on something warm. This stimulates skin respiration and gladu-
lar activity, eliminates harmful substances, toughens the body and
trains the vascular and nervous systems. All types of bathing, regular
baths, steam baths, saunas and swimming are healthful if they are
done in moderation.

b) Fresh air

The healing effects of correct breathing are being recognized now
more than ever. However, breathing can only be done correctly if
abdominal organs are not irritated, as this hampers abdominal
breathing and makes it shallow, which is very common today. *Im-*

proving the condition of the digestive tract with convalescent therapy is therefore a prerequisite for breathing correctly!

It is generally recognized that daily exercise outdoors, keeping a few windows open during the day and night — as long as the purity and temperature of the air outside allow it — and constant circulation of fresh air in the bedroom are all desirable. Nothing can replace a good brisk walk every day! Skin respiration is also encouraged by exposing the body to fresh air in as little clothing as possible, for instance when washing in the morning. Generally speaking, clothing should never impede skin respiration. Tight clothes or clothes made of non-breathable materials, like rubber jackets, shoes, and soles, or the very popular synthetic-fiber garments, like shirts, undershirts, bras, and underwear, made from nylon, perlon, orlon, etc. are not considered good for one's health.

3. Training

Those whose physical activity is either insufficient or limited to one activity need, if they are in relatively good health, compatible physical conditioning.

A daily exercise program of any kind, done with windows open and in light clothing cannot be highly enough recommended. Any moderate involvement in sports, regular exercise in a gym, aerobics, yoga, hiking, walking whenever possible, all types of movement, if not concentrated on one activity, condition the body physically. According to ancient philosophy, life is "self movement", of which the continuous use of one's muscles is also a part. Therefore:

Don't let your body go, exercise it systematically! He who rests, rusts!

A healthier tomorrow

Kings and governments are more easily overthrown than eating habits. It takes knowledge and will power to recognize the full meaning and import of various attitudes — attitudes that have become so ingrained they have practically turned into flesh and blood — and to be able to draw conclusions from them.

Anyone who has gone through Dr. *Mayr*'s cleansing therapy will, from his own experience, have complete sympathy for what has been described here. Others may be less convinced, though they too may have picked up some practical hints. But more than anything, they will not be able to ignore the following facts, and these will be very valuable to them in the future:

1. It is necessary for everyone to do something now and then to maintain or improve his health, without waiting for pain to strike —
2. Prevention is better and easier than a cure —
3. We cannot buy good health with medications, even the most expensive ones —
4. A physician can never give us good health; we earn it ourselves either by our own efforts or by working together with a physician —
5. We cannot achieve any basic improvement in our health as long as we still maintain bad habits —
6. Life styles and eating habits largely determine our physical condition; it depends on us whether our health goes one way or the other —
7. Eating a lot does not make us strong and healthy; it makes us sick, unattractive and prematurely old —
8. The digestive system of the average person is overloaded and contaminated with debris that causes illness —
9. It is therefore necessary to undergo inner cleansing and digestive regeneration treatment from time to time —
10. This therapy prevents a whole range of illnesses, pain and premature aging and restores the body and mind —

If these concepts are understood, their logic cannot be escaped, and some day — sooner or later — everyone will come to the firm resolution:

A healthier tomorrow
means
respite, cleansing and training

References

BARTUSSEK, A.: Darm, Ernährung und Gesundheit. Drei Eichen Verlag, München (1954).

—,—: Das Problem der Ernährung in vertiefter Sicht. Ehk. 5/1956. fahrungsheilkunde 5/1956.

—,—: Diagnostik der Gesundheit nach F. X. Mayr. Ehk 6/1956.

—,—: Dünndarmhypotonie als Grundphänomen der Gesundheitsschädigung. Ehk. 7/1956.

—,—: Grundsätzliches über die Mayr-Kur. Ehk. 2/1981.

—,—: Therapie der Dünndarmhypotonie nach F. X. Mayr. Ehk. 8/1956.

—,—: Zentrale Bedeutung des Dünndarms für Gesundheit und Krankheit. Die Heilkunst 9/1955, Heilkunst-Verlag GmbH, München.

—,—: Mayr-Diät und Behandlung. Die Heilkunst 2/1961.

—,—: Ernährung und Haltung. Die Heilkunst 1/1961.

—,—: Beziehungen zwischen Körperhaltung und Gesundheit. Eutonie. Karl F. Haug Verlag, Heidelberg (1964).

—,—: Die Gesundheitslehre F. X. Mayrs. Der Landarzt 23/1966. Hippokrates-Verlag GmbH, Stuttgart.

—,—: Abwehr von Umweltschäden nach F. X. Mayr. Ehk. 5/1972.

—,—: Das Enteropathie-Syndrom nach F. X. Mayr und der rheumatische Formenkreis. Ehk. 10/73.

—,—: Der chronische Darmschaden. Diagnostik der Gesundheit und Therapie nach F. X. Mayr. W. Braumüller, Univ. Verlag GmbH, Wien (1974).

BECHER, E.: Intestinale Autointoxikation. Ergebnisse der gesamten Medizin 18/1933. Urban & Schwarzenberg KG, Wien.

BRAUCHLE, A.: Naturheilkunde des praktischen Arztes (I und II). Hippokrates-Verlag GmbH, Stuttgart (1951).

—,—: Das große Buch der Naturheilkunde. Mosaik Verlag, Gütersloh (1957).

BUCHINGER, O.: Das Heilfasten. Hippokrates-Verlag GmbH, Stuttgart.

BUCHINGER, O. jun.: Überlegungen zur Fastenkur. Ehk. 5/1978.

DOERFLER, J.: F. X. MAYR-Kur und hämatogene Oxydationstherapie. Ehk. 8/1977.

—,—: HOT — F. X. MAYR-Kur — Symbioselenkung. Ehk. 8/1978.

—,—: Warum ist die MAYR-Kur eine Basistherapie? Ehk. 3/1979.

EMPFENZEDER, K.: Der Kreuzschmerz. Wesen und Behandlung aus der Sicht F. X. Mayrs. Ehk. 11/1970.

—,—: Probleme bei pathologischer Haltung und Gangart. Orthopädische Praxis 7/1974. Medizinisch Literarische Verlags-GmbH, Uelzen.

—,—: Probleme beim Bauchhebegriff. Orthopädische Praxis 8/1976. Medizinisch Literarische Verlags-GmbH, Uelzen.

—,—: Die pathologische Gangart beim genuvalgum. Ursache und Behandlung (nach F. X. MAYR). Ehk. 5/1973.

FELBERMAYR, L.: Herzkrankheiten und Verdauungsapparat. Verlag Neues Leben 5/1955. Bad Goisern.

FREIWALD, E.: Behandlung recid. Ulcera v. et d. mit der Mayr-Kur. Ehk. 8/1982.

—,—: Vermiedene Operationen durch Mayr-Kur. Ehk. 5/1981.

—,—: Migränebehandlung mit der Mayr-Kur. Ehk. 12/1983.

GUGGI, F.: Der Weichteil- oder chemische Rheumatismus. W. Maudrich, Wien (1956).

GUTZEIT, K.: Über die Gastroenteritis. Lehmann, München (1953).

HAMMER, E.: Kosmetik, Schönheit und Verdauung. Kosmetikerinnen-Fachzeitung 311/VII/1978. Baden-Baden.

HEUN, E.: Das Fasten als Erlebnis und Geschehnis. V. Klostermann, Frankfurt/M. (1953).

HOLTZMANN, H. G.: Die Unterschiede der Fastenkuren nach Buchinger und Mayr. Ehk. 5/1978.

KIMMERLE, P. E.: Mayr-Kur und Risikofaktoren. Ehk. 9/1981

KÖHNLECHNER, M.: Handbuch der Naturheilkunde. Kindler Verlag GmbH, München (1975).

KOJER, E.: Grundzüge der Mayrschen Behandlungsmethode. Verlag Neues Leben, 5/1955, Bad Goisern.

—,—: Diagnostik der Gesundheit nach F. X. Mayr. Ehk. 5/1960.

—,—: Ambulante Sanierung des Magen-Darm-Kanals nach F. X. Mayr. Ehk. 4/1969.

—,—: Grundsätzliches zur Therapie nach F. X. Mayr. Ehk. 11/1982

KOJER, E. und Mitarb.: Festschrift zum 100. Geburtstag von Dr. F. X. Mayr. Karl F. Haug Verlag, Heidelberg (1975).

KOJER, M.: Altersdiabetes und Mayr-Kur. Ehk. 6/1983

—,—: Wasserhaushalt und Elektrolyte. Ehk. 7/1982.

KÖTSCHAU, K.: Medizin am Scheideweg. Karl F. Haug Verlag, Heidelberg (1960).

—,—: Gesundheitsprobleme unserer Zeit. H. G. Müller Verlag, Krailling (1955).

MAYR, F. X.: Fundamente zur Diagnostik der Verdauungskrankheiten (1921), Neuauflage Turm-Verlag, Verlagsgemeinschaft F. Zluhan, Bietigheim (1974).

—,—: Die Darmträgheit. 3. Aufl. Verlag Neues Leben, Bad Goisern (1954).

—,—: Die verhängnisvollste Frage. Verlag Neues Leben, Bad Goisern (1951).

—,—: Schönheit und Verdauung. Verlag Neues Leben, Bad Goisern (1954).

MORDHORST, G.: Ableitung über die Haut zur Unterstützung von Regenerationskuren. Ehk. 6/1967, Beilage Diaita.

—,—: Einfache Maßnahmen der physikalischen Therapie zur Unterstützung der Nachbehandlung von Regenerationskuren (F. X. Mayr). Ehk. 1968.

NOTNAGEL, H.: Diagnostik und Therapie der Verdauungskrankheiten. Leipzig (1898).

POLLAK, K.: Der Naturarzt (Kapitel F. X. MAYR-Kur) 1953. Sammlung lebendige Medizin.

PREUSSER, W.: Diagn. u. therap. Nutzung cutivisc. Reflexe b. d. Mayr-Kur. Ehk. 10/1983.

PUTZAR-EHRENBERG, Ch.: Erfahrungen mit der Darmbehandlung nach F. X. Mayr. 22/1963, Hippokrates-Verlag GmbH, Stuttgart.

—,—: Koprolyse durch Fastenkuren. Ärztliches Mitteilungsblatt 8/1950, Berlin.

RAUCH, E.: La depurazione dell' Intestino secondo il Dr. F. X. Mayr. Italienische Übersetzung von Dr. G. BERTOLINI, Selbstverlag, Milano.

—,—: De Darmreinigung folgens Dr. F. X. Mayr. Holländische Übersetzung, De Driehoek, Amsterdam (1976).

—,—: **Blut- und Säftereinigung. Milde Ableitungskur. 13. Aufl., Karl F. Haug Verlag, Heidelberg (1980).**

—,—: Falsches Zitieren F. X. Mayrs. Hippokrates-Verlag GmbH, Stuttgart, 12/1958.

—,—: Der chronische Verdauungsschaden und seine Auswirkungen. Ehk. 3/1958.
—,—: Mayr-Kur in der Großstadtpraxis. Ehk. 5/1970.
—,—: Einfache Schnelldiagnostik von Magen-, Leber-, Dünndarmschäden (Die Succussionen). Ehk. 10/1969.
—,—: Mayr-Kur und Gravidität. Ehk. 11/1973.
—,—: Behandlung akuter Infekte im Sinne F. X. Mayrs. Ehk. 10/1972.
—,—: Heilung der Erkältungs- und Infektionskrankheiten durch natürliche Behandlung. 10. Aufl., Karl F. Haug Verlag, Heidelberg (1980).
—,—: Genezing van verkoudheid en infectieziekten. Holländische Übersetzung, De Driehoek, Amsterdam.
—,—: Aspekte zur Vorsorge- und Gesundheitsdiagnostik nach F. X. MAYR. Ehk. 6/1977.
—,—: Diagnostik nach F. X. MAYR. Kriterien des Krankheitsvorfeldes, der Gesundheit und Krankheit. 2. Aufl., Karl F. Haug Verlag, Heidelberg (1979).
—,—: Diagnostik nach F. X. MAYR. — Einführung. Physikal. Medizin u. Rehabilitation. 9/1978. Uelzen. ML-Verlag.
—,—: Zur Psychologie ärztlicher Kurlenkung. Ehk 1/1982.
RECKEWEG, H.-H.: Homotoxikologie. Aurelia- Verlag, Baden-Baden (1975).
REGAMEY, P. R., OP.: Wiederentdeckung des Fastens. Herold, Wien (1963).
ROST, A.: Der Darm als Störfeld in der thermischen Diagnostik. Ehk. 12/1983.
RUSCH, H. P.: Naturwissenschaft von morgen. H. G. Müller Verlag, Krailling (1955).
—,—: Bodenfruchtbarkeit. 4. Aufl., Karl F. Haug Verlag, Heidelberg (1980).
SALMANOFF, A.: Geheimnisvolle Weisheit des Leibes. Karl F. Haug Verlag, Heidelberg (1961).
SCHMIEDECKER, K.: Untrügliche Zeichen der Gesundheit. Verlag Neues Leben, Bad Goisern (1955).
—,—: Über den Leberbuckel. Medizinische Klinik 19/1958, Urban & Schwarzenberg, München-Berlin.
—,—: Gesundung und ihr Training. Verlag Neues Leben, Bad Goisern (1970).
SCHMITZ-HARBAUER, R.: Raucherentwöhnungshilfe durch Kostumstellung. Münchner Med. Wochenschrift 11/1974.
STEFAN, K.: Abbau und Aufbau als Heilprinzip. Karl F. Haug Verlag, Heidelberg (1958).
SOBOTIK, S.: Schonkost — Diätkost. Verlag Neues Leben, 6/1954, Bad Goisern.
—,—: Bircher-Benner — F. X. MAYR. Verlag Neues Leben, Bad Goisern 1955.
TRUDEL, E.: Die ambulante MAYR-Kur. Ehk. 12/1977.
—,—: Behandlung scheinbarer Psychopathien mit der Mayr-Kur. Ehk. 9/1981.
—,—: Behandlung chronischer Entzündungszustände im Unterbauch (chron. Prostatitis und Adnexitis) Ehk. 7/1984.
VOGEL-HAFERKAMP: Biologisch-medizinisches Taschenjahrbuch 56/1955. Hippokrates-Verlag GmbH, Stuttgart.
WOLFRUM, W.: Aktive Gesundheitspflege nach F. X. Mayr. Bietigheim, Turm-Verlag.
—,—: Mayr-Kur und Obstipation. Ehk. 5/1979.
—,—: Die Mayr-Kur. Österr. Ärztezeitung 36/6, 1981, Wien.
—,—: Behandlung von Alterskrankheiten nach Mayr. Ehk. 9/1981.
—,—: Gesunde Ernährung aus der Sicht F. X. Mayrs. Ehk. 12/1983.
ZABEL, W.: Das Fasten. Hippokrates-Verlag GmbH, Stuttgart (1962).